Mometrix
TEST PREPARATION

AF901630

Secrets of the ARDMS®

Adult Echocardiography Exam Study Guide

Dear Future Exam Success Story

First of all, **THANK YOU** for purchasing Mometrix study materials!

Second, congratulations! You are one of the few determined test-takers who are committed to doing whatever it takes to excel on your exam. **You have come to the right place.** We developed these study materials with one goal in mind: to deliver you the information you need in a format that's concise and easy to use.

In addition to optimizing your guide for the content of the test, we've outlined our recommended steps for breaking down the preparation process into small, attainable goals so you can make sure you stay on track.

We've also analyzed the entire test-taking process, identifying the most common pitfalls and showing how you can overcome them and be ready for any curveball the test throws you.

Standardized testing is one of the biggest obstacles on your road to success, which only increases the importance of doing well in the high-pressure, high-stakes environment of test day. Your results on this test could have a significant impact on your future, and this guide provides the information and practical advice to help you achieve your full potential on test day.

Your success is our success

We would love to hear from you! If you would like to share the story of your exam success or if you have any questions or comments in regard to our products, please contact us at **800-673-8175** or **support@mometrix.com**.

Thanks again for your business and we wish you continued success!

Sincerely,
The Mometrix Test Preparation Team

Need more help? Check out our flashcards at:
http://MometrixFlashcards.com/ARDMS

Written and edited by the Mometrix Exam Secrets Test Prep Team
Printed in the United States of America

TABLE OF CONTENTS

INTRODUCTION 1
SECRET KEY 1: PLAN BIG, STUDY SMALL 2
SECRET KEY 2: MAKE YOUR STUDYING COUNT 4
SECRET KEY 3: PRACTICE THE RIGHT WAY 6
SECRET KEY 4: PACE YOURSELF 8
SECRET KEY 5: HAVE A PLAN FOR GUESSING 10
TEST-TAKING STRATEGIES 13
ANATOMY AND PHYSIOLOGY 19
PATHOLOGY 26
CLINICAL CARE AND SAFETY 49
MEASUREMENT TECHNIQUES, MANEUVERS, AND SONOGRAPHIC VIEWS 52
INSTRUMENTATION, OPTIMIZATION, AND CONTRAST 62
HOW TO OVERCOME TEST ANXIETY 68
ONLINE RESOURCES 75

Introduction

Thank you for purchasing this resource! You have made the choice to prepare yourself for a test that could have a huge impact on your future, and this guide is designed to help you be fully ready for test day. Obviously, it's important to have a solid understanding of the test material, but you also need to be prepared for the unique environment and stressors of the test, so that you can perform to the best of your abilities.

For this purpose, the first section that appears in this guide is the **Secret Keys**. We've devoted countless hours to meticulously researching what works and what doesn't, and we've boiled down our findings to the five most impactful steps you can take to improve your performance on the test. We start at the beginning with study planning and move through the preparation process, all the way to the testing strategies that will help you get the most out of what you know when you're finally sitting in front of the test.

We recommend that you start preparing for your test as far in advance as possible. However, if you've bought this guide as a last-minute study resource and only have a few days before your test, we recommend that you skip over the first two Secret Keys since they address a long-term study plan.

If you struggle with **test anxiety**, we strongly encourage you to check out our recommendations for how you can overcome it. Test anxiety is a formidable foe, but it can be beaten, and we want to make sure you have the tools you need to defeat it.

Secret Key 1: Plan Big, Study Small

There's a lot riding on your performance. If you want to ace this test, you're going to need to keep your skills sharp and the material fresh in your mind. You need a plan that lets you review everything you need to know while still fitting in your schedule. We'll break this strategy down into three categories.

Information Organization

Start with the information you already have: the official test outline. From this, you can make a complete list of all the concepts you need to cover before the test. Organize these concepts into groups that can be studied together, and create a list of any related vocabulary you need to learn so you can brush up on any difficult terms. You'll want to keep this vocabulary list handy once you actually start studying since you may need to add to it along the way.

Time Management

Once you have your set of study concepts, decide how to spread them out over the time you have left before the test. Break your study plan into small, clear goals so you have a manageable task for each day and know exactly what you're doing. Then just focus on one small step at a time. When you manage your time this way, you don't need to spend hours at a time studying. Studying a small block of content for a short period each day helps you retain information better and avoid stressing over how much you have left to do. You can relax knowing that you have a plan to cover everything in time. In order for this strategy to be effective though, you have to start studying early and stick to your schedule. Avoid the exhaustion and futility that comes from last-minute cramming!

Study Environment

The environment you study in has a big impact on your learning. Studying in a coffee shop, while probably more enjoyable, is not likely to be as fruitful as studying in a quiet room. It's important to keep distractions to a minimum. You're only planning to study for a short block of time, so make the most of it. Don't pause to check your phone or get up to find a snack. It's also important to **avoid multitasking**. Research has consistently shown that multitasking will make your studying dramatically less effective. Your study area should also be comfortable and well-lit so you don't have the distraction of straining your eyes or sitting on an uncomfortable chair.

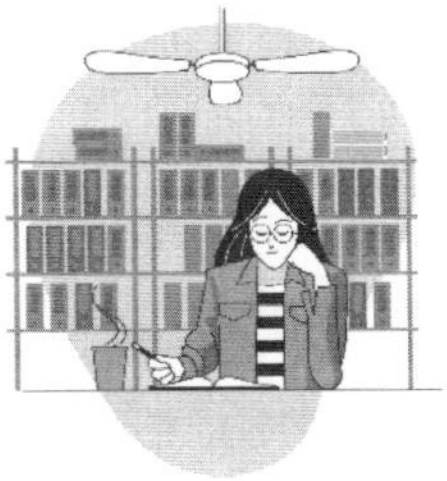

The time of day you study is also important. You want to be rested and alert. Don't wait until just before bedtime. Study when you'll be most likely to comprehend and remember. Even better, if you know what time of day your test will be, set that time aside for study. That way your brain will be used to working on that subject at that specific time and you'll have a better chance of recalling information.

Finally, it can be helpful to team up with others who are studying for the same test. Your actual studying should be done in as isolated an environment as possible, but the work of organizing the information and setting up the study plan can be divided up. In between study sessions, you can discuss with your teammates the concepts that you're all studying and quiz each other on the details. Just be sure that your teammates are as serious about the test as you are. If you find that your study time is being replaced with social time, you might need to find a new team.

Secret Key 2: Make Your Studying Count

You're devoting a lot of time and effort to preparing for this test, so you want to be absolutely certain it will pay off. This means doing more than just reading the content and hoping you can remember it on test day. It's important to make every minute of study count. There are two main areas you can focus on to make your studying count.

Retention

It doesn't matter how much time you study if you can't remember the material. You need to make sure you are retaining the concepts. To check your retention of the information you're learning, try recalling it at later times with minimal prompting. Try carrying around flashcards and glance at one or two from time to time or ask a friend who's also studying for the test to quiz you.

To enhance your retention, look for ways to put the information into practice so that you can apply it rather than simply recalling it. If you're using the information in practical ways, it will be much easier to remember. Similarly, it helps to solidify a concept in your mind if you're not only reading it to yourself but also explaining it to someone else. Ask a friend to let you teach them about a concept you're a little shaky on (or speak aloud to an imaginary audience if necessary). As you try to summarize, define, give examples, and answer your friend's questions, you'll understand the concepts better and they will stay with you longer. Finally, step back for a big picture view and ask yourself how each piece of information fits with the whole subject. When you link the different concepts together and see them working together as a whole, it's easier to remember the individual components.

Finally, practice showing your work on any multi-step problems, even if you're just studying. Writing out each step you take to solve a problem will help solidify the process in your mind, and you'll be more likely to remember it during the test.

Modality

Modality simply refers to the means or method by which you study. Choosing a study modality that fits your own individual learning style is crucial. No two people learn best in exactly the same way, so it's important to know your strengths and use them to your advantage.

For example, if you learn best by visualization, focus on visualizing a concept in your mind and draw an image or a diagram. Try color-coding your notes, illustrating them, or creating symbols that will trigger your mind to recall a learned concept. If you learn best by hearing or discussing information, find a study partner who learns the same way or read aloud to yourself. Think about how to put the information in your own words. Imagine that you are giving a lecture on the topic and record yourself so you can listen to it later.

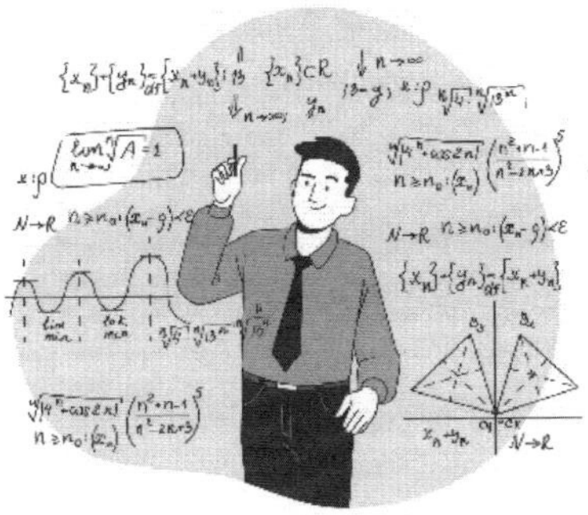

For any learning style, flashcards can be helpful. Organize the information so you can take advantage of spare moments to review. Underline key words or phrases. Use different colors for different categories. Mnemonic devices (such as creating a short list in which every item starts with the same letter) can also help with retention. Find what works best for you and use it to store the information in your mind most effectively and easily.

Secret Key 3: Practice the Right Way

Your success on test day depends not only on how many hours you put into preparing, but also on whether you prepared the right way. It's good to check along the way to see if your studying is paying off. One of the most effective ways to do this is by taking practice tests to evaluate your progress. Practice tests are useful because they show exactly where you need to improve. Every time you take a practice test, pay special attention to these three groups of questions:

- The questions you got wrong
- The questions you had to guess on, even if you guessed right
- The questions you found difficult or slow to work through

This will show you exactly what your weak areas are, and where you need to devote more study time. Ask yourself why each of these questions gave you trouble. Was it because you didn't understand the material? Was it because you didn't remember the vocabulary? Do you need more repetitions on this type of question to build speed and confidence? Dig into those questions and figure out how you can strengthen your weak areas as you go back to review the material.

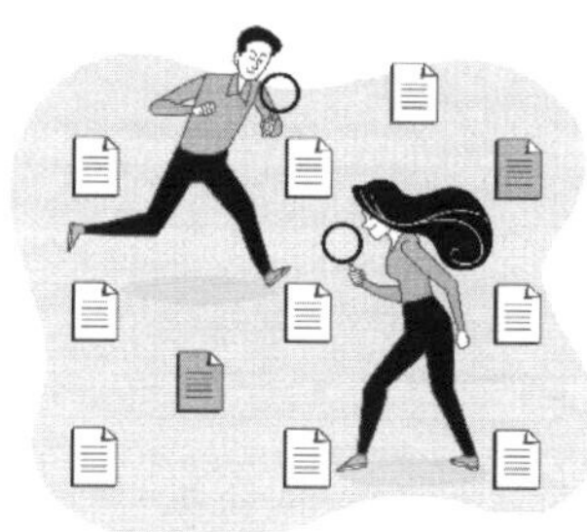

Additionally, many practice tests have a section explaining the answer choices. It can be tempting to read the explanation and think that you now have a good understanding of the concept. However, an explanation likely only covers part of the question's broader context. Even if the explanation makes perfect sense, **go back and investigate** every concept related to the question until you're positive you have a thorough understanding.

As you go along, keep in mind that the practice test is just that: practice. Memorizing these questions and answers will not be very helpful on the actual test because it is unlikely to have any of the same exact questions. If you only know the right answers to the sample questions, you won't be prepared for the real thing. **Study the concepts** until you understand them fully, and then you'll be able to answer any question that shows up on the test.

It's important to wait on the practice tests until you're ready. If you take a test on your first day of study, you may be overwhelmed by the amount of material covered and how much you need to learn. Work up to it gradually.

On test day, you'll need to be prepared for answering questions, managing your time, and using the test-taking strategies you've learned. It's a lot to balance, like a mental marathon that will have a big impact on your future. Like training for a marathon, you'll need to start slowly and work your way up. When test day arrives, you'll be ready.

Start with the strategies you've read in the first two Secret Keys—plan your course and study in the way that works best for you. If you have time, consider using multiple study resources to get different approaches to the same concepts. It can be helpful to see difficult concepts from more than one angle. Then find a good source for practice tests. Many times, the test website will suggest potential study resources or provide sample tests.

Practice Test Strategy

If you're able to find at least three practice tests, we recommend this strategy:

Untimed and Open-Book Practice

Take the first test with no time constraints and with your notes and study guide handy. Take your time and focus on applying the strategies you've learned.

Timed and Open-Book Practice

Take the second practice test open-book as well, but set a timer and practice pacing yourself to finish in time.

Timed and Closed-Book Practice

Take any other practice tests as if it were test day. Set a timer and put away your study materials. Sit at a table or desk in a quiet room, imagine yourself at the testing center, and answer questions as quickly and accurately as possible.

Keep repeating timed and closed-book tests on a regular basis until you run out of practice tests or it's time for the actual test. Your mind will be ready for the schedule and stress of test day, and you'll be able to focus on recalling the material you've learned.

Secret Key 4: Pace Yourself

Once you're fully prepared for the material on the test, your biggest challenge on test day will be managing your time. Just knowing that the clock is ticking can make you panic even if you have plenty of time left. Work on pacing yourself so you can build confidence against the time constraints of the exam. Pacing is a difficult skill to master, especially in a high-pressure environment, so **practice is vital**.

Set time expectations for your pace based on how much time is available. For example, if a section has 60 questions and the time limit is 30 minutes, you know you have to average 30 seconds or less per question in order to answer them all. Although 30 seconds is the hard limit, set 25 seconds per question as your goal, so you reserve extra time to spend on harder questions. When you budget extra time for the harder questions, you no longer have any reason to stress when those questions take longer to answer.

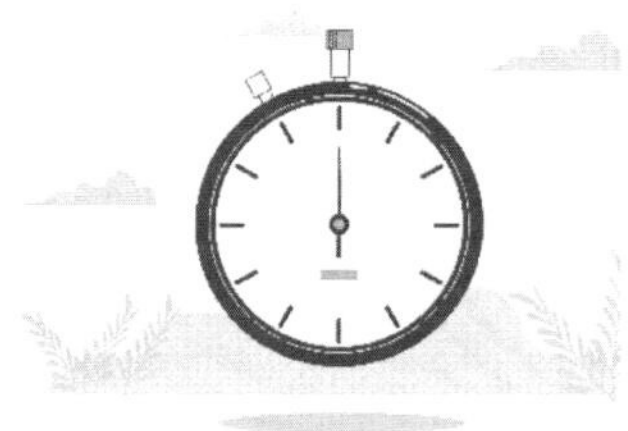

Don't let this time expectation distract you from working through the test at a calm, steady pace, but keep it in mind so you don't spend too much time on any one question. Recognize that taking extra time on one question you don't understand may keep you from answering two that you do understand later in the test. If your time limit for a question is up and you're still not sure of the answer, mark it and move on, and come back to it later if the time and the test format allow. If the testing format doesn't allow you to return to earlier questions, just make an educated guess; then put it out of your mind and move on.

On the easier questions, be careful not to rush. It may seem wise to hurry through them so you have more time for the challenging ones, but it's not worth missing one if you know the concept and just didn't take the time to read the question fully. Work efficiently but make sure you understand the question and have looked at all of the answer choices, since more than one may seem right at first.

Even if you're paying attention to the time, you may find yourself a little behind at some point. You should speed up to get back on track, but do so wisely. Don't panic; just take a few seconds less on each question until you're caught up. Don't guess without thinking, but do look through the answer choices and eliminate any you know are wrong. If you can get down to two choices, it is often worthwhile to guess from those. Once you've chosen an answer, move on and don't dwell on any that you skipped or had to hurry through. If a question was taking too long, chances are it was one of the harder ones, so you weren't as likely to get it right anyway.

On the other hand, if you find yourself getting ahead of schedule, it may be beneficial to slow down a little. The more quickly you work, the more likely you are to make a careless mistake that will affect your score. You've budgeted time for each question, so don't be afraid to spend that time. Practice an efficient but careful pace to get the most out of the time you have.

Secret Key 5: Have a Plan for Guessing

When you're taking the test, you may find yourself stuck on a question. Some of the answer choices seem better than others, but you don't see the one answer choice that is obviously correct. What do you do?

The scenario described above is very common, yet most test takers have not effectively prepared for it. Developing and practicing a plan for guessing may be one of the single most effective uses of your time as you get ready for the exam.

In developing your plan for guessing, there are three questions to address:

- When should you start the guessing process?
- How should you narrow down the choices?
- Which answer should you choose?

When to Start the Guessing Process

Unless your plan for guessing is to select C every time (which, despite its merits, is not what we recommend), you need to leave yourself enough time to apply your answer elimination strategies. Since you have a limited amount of time for each question, that means that if you're going to give yourself the best shot at guessing correctly, you have to decide quickly whether or not you will guess.

Of course, the best-case scenario is that you don't have to guess at all, so first, see if you can answer the question based on your knowledge of the subject and basic reasoning skills. Focus on the key words in the question and try to jog your memory of related topics. Give yourself a chance to bring the knowledge to mind, but once you realize that you don't have (or you can't access) the knowledge you need to answer the question, it's time to start the guessing process.

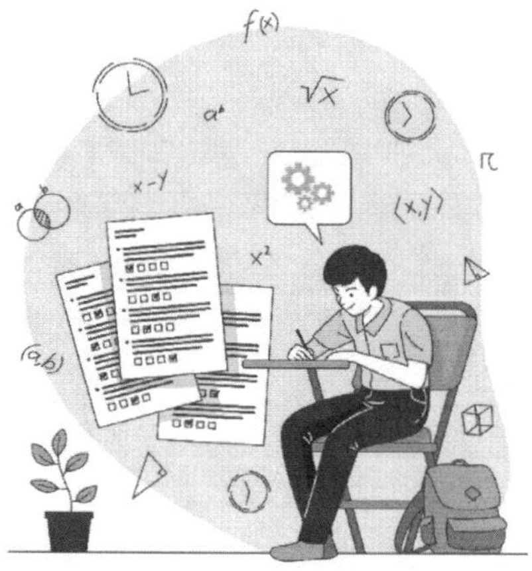

It's almost always better to start the guessing process too early than too late. It only takes a few seconds to remember something and answer the question from knowledge. Carefully eliminating wrong answer choices takes longer. Plus, going through the process of eliminating answer choices can actually help jog your memory.

Summary: Start the guessing process as soon as you decide that you can't answer the question based on your knowledge.

How to Narrow Down the Choices

The next chapter in this book (**Test-Taking Strategies**) includes a wide range of strategies for how to approach questions and how to look for answer choices to eliminate. You will definitely want to read those carefully, practice them, and figure out which ones work best for you. Here though, we're going to address a mindset rather than a particular strategy.

Your odds of guessing an answer correctly depend on how many options you are choosing from.

Number of options left	5	4	3	2	1
Odds of guessing correctly	20%	25%	33%	50%	100%

You can see from this chart just how valuable it is to be able to eliminate incorrect answers and make an educated guess, but there are two things that many test takers do that cause them to miss out on the benefits of guessing:

- Accidentally eliminating the correct answer
- Selecting an answer based on an impression

We'll look at the first one here, and the second one in the next section.

To avoid accidentally eliminating the correct answer, we recommend a thought exercise called **the $5 challenge**. In this challenge, you only eliminate an answer choice from contention if you are willing to bet $5 on it being wrong. Why $5? Five dollars is a small but not insignificant amount of money. It's an amount you could afford to lose but wouldn't want to throw away. And while losing $5 once might not hurt too much, doing it twenty times will set you back $100. In the same way, each small decision you make—eliminating a choice here, guessing on a question there—won't by itself impact your score very much, but when you put them all together, they can make a big difference. By holding each answer choice elimination decision to a higher standard, you can reduce the risk of accidentally eliminating the correct answer.

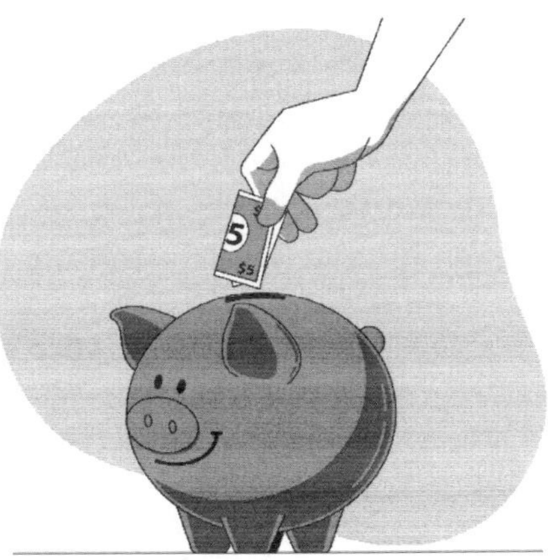

The $5 challenge can also be applied in a positive sense: If you are willing to bet $5 that an answer choice *is* correct, go ahead and mark it as correct.

Summary: Only eliminate an answer choice if you are willing to bet $5 that it is wrong.

Which Answer to Choose

You're taking the test. You've run into a hard question and decided you'll have to guess. You've eliminated all the answer choices you're willing to bet $5 on. Now you have to pick an answer. Why do we even need to talk about this? Why can't you just pick whichever one you feel like when the time comes?

The answer to these questions is that if you don't come into the test with a plan, you'll rely on your impression to select an answer choice, and if you do that, you risk falling into a trap. The test writers know that everyone who takes their test will be guessing on some of the questions, so they intentionally write wrong answer choices to seem plausible. You still have to pick an answer though, and if the wrong answer choices are designed to look right, how can you ever be sure that you're not falling for their trap? The best solution we've found to this dilemma is to take the decision out of your hands entirely. Here is the process we recommend:

Once you've eliminated any choices that you are confident (willing to bet $5) are wrong, select the first remaining choice as your answer.

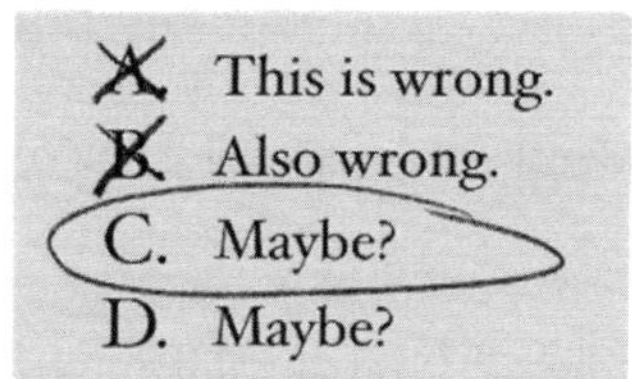

Whether you choose to select the first remaining choice, the second, or the last, the important thing is that you use some preselected standard. Using this approach guarantees that you will not be enticed into selecting an answer choice that looks right, because you are not basing your decision on how the answer choices look.

This is not meant to make you question your knowledge. Instead, it is to help you recognize the difference between your knowledge and your impressions. There's a huge difference between thinking an answer is right because of what you know, and thinking an answer is right because it looks or sounds like it should be right.

Summary: To ensure that your selection is appropriately random, make a predetermined selection from among all answer choices you have not eliminated.

Test-Taking Strategies

This section contains a list of test-taking strategies that you may find helpful as you work through the test. By taking what you know and applying logical thought, you can maximize your chances of answering any question correctly!

It is very important to realize that every question is different and every person is different: no single strategy will work on every question, and no single strategy will work for every person. That's why we've included all of them here, so you can try them out and determine which ones work best for different types of questions and which ones work best for you.

Question Strategies

✓ Read Carefully

Read the question and the answer choices carefully. Don't miss the question because you misread the terms. You have plenty of time to read each question thoroughly and make sure you understand what is being asked. Yet a happy medium must be attained, so don't waste too much time. You must read carefully and efficiently.

✓ Contextual Clues

Look for contextual clues. If the question includes a word you are not familiar with, look at the immediate context for some indication of what the word might mean. Contextual clues can often give you all the information you need to decipher the meaning of an unfamiliar word. Even if you can't determine the meaning, you may be able to narrow down the possibilities enough to make a solid guess at the answer to the question.

✓ Prefixes

If you're having trouble with a word in the question or answer choices, try dissecting it. Take advantage of every clue that the word might include. Prefixes can be a huge help. Usually, they allow you to determine a basic meaning. *Pre-* means before, *post-* means after, *pro-* is positive, *de-* is negative. From prefixes, you can get an idea of the general meaning of the word and try to put it into context.

✓ Hedge Words

Watch out for critical hedge words, such as *likely, may, can, often, almost, mostly, usually, generally, rarely,* and *sometimes.* Question writers insert these hedge phrases to cover every possibility. Often an answer choice will be wrong simply because it leaves no room for exception. Be on guard for answer choices that have definitive words such as *exactly* and *always.*

☑ Switchback Words

Stay alert for *switchbacks*. These are the words and phrases frequently used to alert you to shifts in thought. The most common switchback words are *but*, *although*, and *however*. Others include *nevertheless, on the other hand, even though, while, in spite of, despite*, and *regardless of*. Switchback words are important to catch because they can change the direction of the question or an answer choice.

☑ Face Value

When in doubt, use common sense. Accept the situation in the problem at face value. Don't read too much into it. These problems will not require you to make wild assumptions. If you have to go beyond creativity and warp time or space in order to have an answer choice fit the question, then you should move on and consider the other answer choices. These are normal problems rooted in reality. The applicable relationship or explanation may not be readily apparent, but it is there for you to figure out. Use your common sense to interpret anything that isn't clear.

Answer Choice Strategies

☑ Answer Selection

The most thorough way to pick an answer choice is to identify and eliminate wrong answers until only one is left, then confirm it is the correct answer. Sometimes an answer choice may immediately seem right, but be careful. The test writers will usually put more than one reasonable answer choice on each question, so take a second to read all of them and make sure that the other choices are not equally obvious. As long as you have time left, it is better to read every answer choice than to pick the first one that looks right without checking the others.

☑ Answer Choice Families

An answer choice family consists of two (in rare cases, three) answer choices that are very similar in construction and cannot all be true at the same time. If you see two answer choices that are direct opposites or parallels, one of them is usually the correct answer. For instance, if one answer choice says that quantity *x* increases and another either says that quantity *x* decreases (opposite) or says that quantity *y* increases (parallel), then those answer choices would fall into the same family. An answer choice that doesn't match the construction of the answer choice family is more likely to be incorrect. Most questions will not have answer choice families, but when they do appear, you should be prepared to recognize them.

☑ Eliminate Answers

Eliminate answer choices as soon as you realize they are wrong, but make sure you consider all possibilities. If you are eliminating answer choices and realize that the last one you are left with is also wrong, don't panic. Start over and consider each choice again. There may be something you missed the first time that you will realize on the second pass.

⊘ Avoid Fact Traps

Don't be distracted by an answer choice that is factually true but doesn't answer the question. You are looking for the choice that answers the question. Stay focused on what the question is asking for so you don't accidentally pick an answer that is true but incorrect. Always go back to the question and make sure the answer choice you've selected actually answers the question and is not merely a true statement.

⊘ Extreme Statements

In general, you should avoid answers that put forth extreme actions as standard practice or proclaim controversial ideas as established fact. An answer choice that states the "process should be used in certain situations, if..." is much more likely to be correct than one that states the "process should be discontinued completely." The first is a calm rational statement and doesn't even make a definitive, uncompromising stance, using a hedge word *if* to provide wiggle room, whereas the second choice is far more extreme.

⊘ Benchmark

As you read through the answer choices and you come across one that seems to answer the question well, mentally select that answer choice. This is not your final answer, but it's the one that will help you evaluate the other answer choices. The one that you selected is your benchmark or standard for judging each of the other answer choices. Every other answer choice must be compared to your benchmark. That choice is correct until proven otherwise by another answer choice beating it. If you find a better answer, then that one becomes your new benchmark. Once you've decided that no other choice answers the question as well as your benchmark, you have your final answer.

⊘ Predict the Answer

Before you even start looking at the answer choices, it is often best to try to predict the answer. When you come up with the answer on your own, it is easier to avoid distractions and traps because you will know exactly what to look for. The right answer choice is unlikely to be word-for-word what you came up with, but it should be a close match. Even if you are confident that you have the right answer, you should still take the time to read each option before moving on.

General Strategies

⊘ Tough Questions

If you are stumped on a problem or it appears too hard or too difficult, don't waste time. Move on! Remember though, if you can quickly check for obviously incorrect answer choices, your chances of guessing correctly are greatly improved. Before you completely give up, at least try to knock out a couple of possible answers. Eliminate what you can and then guess at the remaining answer choices before moving on.

⊘ Check Your Work

Since you will probably not know every term listed and the answer to every question, it is important that you get credit for the ones that you do know. Don't miss any questions through careless mistakes. If at all possible, try to take a second to look back over your answer selection and make sure you've selected the correct answer choice and haven't made a costly careless mistake (such as marking an answer choice that you didn't mean to mark). This quick double check should more than pay for itself in caught mistakes for the time it costs.

⊘ Pace Yourself

It's easy to be overwhelmed when you're looking at a page full of questions; your mind is confused and full of random thoughts, and the clock is ticking down faster than you would like. Calm down and maintain the pace that you have set for yourself. Especially as you get down to the last few minutes of the test, don't let the small numbers on the clock make you panic. As long as you are on track by monitoring your pace, you are guaranteed to have time for each question.

⊘ Don't Rush

It is very easy to make errors when you are in a hurry. Maintaining a fast pace in answering questions is pointless if it makes you miss questions that you would have gotten right otherwise. Test writers like to include distracting information and wrong answers that seem right. Taking a little extra time to avoid careless mistakes can make all the difference in your test score. Find a pace that allows you to be confident in the answers that you select.

⊘ Keep Moving

Panicking will not help you pass the test, so do your best to stay calm and keep moving. Taking deep breaths and going through the answer elimination steps you practiced can help to break through a stress barrier and keep your pace.

Final Notes

The combination of a solid foundation of content knowledge and the confidence that comes from practicing your plan for applying that knowledge is the key to maximizing your performance on test day. As your foundation of content knowledge is built up and strengthened, you'll find that the strategies included in this chapter become more and more effective in helping you quickly sift through the distractions and traps of the test to isolate the correct answer.

Now that you're preparing to move forward into the test content chapters of this book, be sure to keep your goal in mind. As you read, think about how you will be able to apply this information on the test. If you've already seen sample questions for the test and you have an idea of the question format and style, try to come up with questions of your own that you can answer based on what you're reading. This will give you valuable practice applying your knowledge in the same ways you can expect to on test day.

Good luck and good studying!

Anatomy and Physiology

Cardiac Function and Structures

A normal heart is situated in the left side of the chest, and the bottom of the heart is tethered by the great vessels: the aorta, superior vena cava, and the main pulmonary artery. The apex of the heart is located anterior, inferior, and 60 degrees to the left side. The heart is comprised of two thick-walled ventricles and two thin-walled atria with four valves in between the chambers that function to separate blood flow. Four pulmonary veins drain into the left atrium and serve to fill the left heart by blood flowing through the mitral valve.

The left ventricle has a thick wall and is the biggest of the four chambers of the heart. Blood flows from the left ventricle into the aorta and thus into the systemic circulation. The ascending aorta is called the left ventricular outflow tract and looks similar to a tube on a long axis. The aortic valve is visualized in this plane because the noncoronary cusp leaflet and the right coronary cusp leaflet are shut in diastole and open in systole. The left coronary cusp leaflet may sometimes also be visualized in this view.

Review Video: Heart Blood Flow and Heart Anatomy
Visit mometrix.com/academy and enter code: 783139

Review Video: Mnemonics for Heart Anatomy and Physiology
Visit mometrix.com/academy and enter code: 849489

Review Video: Heart Anatomy and Physiology
Visit mometrix.com/academy and enter code: 569724

Right Heart

The right ventricle is located underneath the sternum and is anterior to the left ventricle. The muscle mass of the right ventricle is about one-sixth that of the left ventricle as it pumps against less resistance. The right ventricle has thin walls and is shaped like a crescent as opposed to the left ventricle, which appears ellipsoid in shape. Two divisions to the right ventricle, the inflow tract and the outflow tract, are divided by the crista supraventricularis. The moderator band is attached to the outflow tract and goes from the septum to the anterior wall of the right ventricle.

Nomenclature for Segmental Wall Motion

The left ventricle is divided into three sections (basal, mid, and apical) along its short axis. The basal and middle sections are subsequently divided into six segments. The apical segment is further divided into four segments with the true apex being designated as a single segment. The basal segments are as follows: basal anterior, basal anteroseptal, basal inferoseptal, basal inferior, basal inferolateral, and basal anterolateral. Midcavity segments are midanterior, midanteroseptal, midinferoseptal, midinferior, midinferolateral, and midanterolateral. Apical segments are apical anterior, apical septal, apical inferior, apical lateral, and apex.

Great Vessels

The veins and arteries that enter and leave the heart are known as the great vessels and include the aorta, superior and inferior vena cava, pulmonary trunk, and pulmonary veins. The superior and inferior vena cava function to return oxygen-depleted blood to the right atrium. The pulmonary trunk (right and left pulmonary arteries) then takes this venous blood from the right ventricle to the lungs where it is oxygenated. Oxygenated blood is deposited into the left atrium and then is pumped into the left ventricle. The aorta transports oxygenated blood from the left ventricle into the systemic circulation.

Heart Valves

Heart valves are true flaps that are situated at the ends of the two ventricles of the heart and serve to prevent a backflow of blood and function as one-way inflow inlets on one side of the ventricle and one-way outflow outlets on the other side of the ventricle. All the valves except for the mitral valve have three flaps; the mitral valve has two flaps. The tricuspid valve is positioned between the right atrium and the right ventricle. The pulmonary valve is between the right ventricle and the pulmonary artery. The mitral valve is between the left atrium and left ventricle, while the aortic valve is between the left ventricle and the aorta.

Coronary Sinus

The coronary sinus is located on the posterior aspect of the coronary sulcus on the back of the heart. The coronary sinus serves to empty into the right atrium directly near the area where the posterior interventricular sulcus and the coronary sulcus (crux cordis) join. This area is situated in between the tricuspid valve and the inferior vena cava. The opening of the coronary sinus may sometimes be covered by a Thebesian valve. Most of the epidural ventricular veins drain into the coronary sinus. The primary function of the coronary sinus is to collect cardiac venous blood.

Pericardial and Pleural Structures

The pericardium is a cone-shaped fibrous and serous sac that holds the heart and the great vessels. The pericardium is located in the mediastinum behind the sternum and the cartilages of the left-sided third through seventh ribs. The pericardium is comprised of two closely associated sacs; the outer sac is the fibrous pericardium, and the inner sac is the serous pericardium. The fibrous pericardium fuses with the outer layers of the great vessels and is attached at the base to the central tendon and muscles of the left side of the diaphragm.

Aortic Arch

The aortic arch is the aspect of the aorta that originates at the right-sided second intercostal articulation and traverses initially upward, backward, and then to the left anterior to the trachea. The aortic arch then runs backward at the left side of the trachea and distally on the left side of the fourth thoracic vertebra wherein the arch becomes contiguous with the descending aorta. The aortic arch is located within the mediastinum. The aortic arch may vary in height from as high as the third thoracic vertebra to as low as the fifth thoracic vertebra. The arch of the aorta is composed of three layers: (1) the intima, which functions as a smooth surface for blood flow, (2) the media, which enables expansion and contraction with the heartbeat, and (3) the adventitia, which functions to provide support and structure to the aortic arch.

Inferior and Superior Vena Cava and Hepatic Veins

The superior vena cava and the inferior vena cava function to return deoxygenated blood from the body to the right atrium. The superior vena cava empties deoxygenated blood into the right atrium from the brain, head, neck, upper extremities, and thoracic wall. The inferior vena cava empties deoxygenated blood into the right atrium from the abdomen, pelvis, and lower extremities. The portal venous system originates in capillaries in the walls of the digestive tract (stomach to the rectum) and terminates in capillaries in the liver. Portal venous blood exits the liver via the hepatic veins, which then empty into the inferior vena cava.

Electrical Atrial Systole

Electrical cardiac systole is initiated via a sympathetic charge derived from the sinoatrial (SA) node. From the SA node, the charge travels through the atrial mass to the atrioventricular (AV) node. Atrial systole refers to the contraction of the left and right atrial myocardium. The cells of the SA node are excited electrically when the membranes are depolarized above the excitation threshold. At this stage, voltage-gated calcium channels located on the membranes of the cells open and facilitate the passage of calcium ions into the sarcoplasm of the myocardial cells, which bind to troponin C to cause cross-bridge cycling. Cross-bridge cycling serves to aid in the spread of the cardiac action potential.

Review Video: Electrical Conduction System of the Heart
Visit mometrix.com/academy and enter code: 624557

Mechanical Atrial Systole

Electrical systole functions to open the sodium, potassium, and calcium channels. The elevation in calcium stimulates the interplay between actin and myosin with adenosine triphosphate (ATP) to generate force. Atrial systole happens in late ventricular diastole as a result of the decreased pressure in the ventricles that occurs during ventricular diastole. The decrease in ventricular pressure functions to open the atrioventricular valves and facilitates the passage of blood from the atria into the ventricles. Systole of the right atrium is in conjunction with right ventricular diastole, while left atrial systole occurs in conjunction with left ventricular diastole.

Electrical Systole in the Ventricles

The sinoatrial node creates an electrical signal, which is then spread to the ventricles. The spread of electrical activity to the ventricles is facilitated via the following conducting pathways: internodal pathways and atrial fibers, the atrioventricular node, right and left branches of the bundle of His, and Purkinje fibers. The electrical impulse from the SA node travels to the AV node by means of the internodal fibers; there is a 0.2-second delay while the atria contract. After the delay, the impulse is sent to the ventricles via the bundle of His and the Purkinje fibers, which results in ventricular contraction.

Mechanical Ventricular Systole

Ventricular systole is the contraction of the left and right ventricles. Ventricular systole causes an increase in pressure in the left and right ventricles; when the ventricular pressure exceeds that of the atria, the tricuspid and mitral valves close. Isovolumetric contraction allows the pressure in the ventricles to continue to elevate until maximum pressure generation occurs (max dP/dt). At maximum pressure generation, the pulmonary and aortic valves open to begin the ejection phase. During the ejection phase, blood flows via a pressure gradient through the aorta and pulmonary artery from the left and right ventricles.

Electrical and Mechanical Diastole

Atrial diastole occurs after atrial systole and during ventricular systole. When the left atrium relaxes, it is filled with blood from the pulmonary veins; the right atrium relaxes and is filled with blood from the superior and inferior vena cavae. When the ventricles repolarize, ventricular diastole occurs. The decrease in ventricular pressure below the atrial pressure opens the mitral and tricuspid valves to facilitate blood from the atria that accumulated during systole to rapidly fill the ventricles (rapid ventricular filling). The continued ventricular relaxation serves to draw more blood from the atria. Diastole diminishes as the pressures in the atria and ventricles equalize.

Phases of the Cardiac Cycle

The cardiac cycle may be divided into two basic phases: systole and diastole. Systole is representative of the time period in which the left and right ventricles contract and thus eject blood into the aorta and pulmonary artery. Because the atrioventricular valves are shut during systole, no blood fills the ventricles but it continues to fill the atria. Diastole is representative of ventricular relaxation. The cardiac cycle is typically divided into seven phases as follows: atrial contraction, isovolumetric contraction, rapid ejection, reduced ejection, isovolumetric relaxation, rapid filling, and reduced filling.

Atrial Contraction (Phase 1)

Phase 1 of the cardiac cycle is atrial contraction, wherein the atrioventricular (AV) valves are open, and the semilunar (SL) valves are closed. Phase 1 originates with the electrical depolarization of the atria, which serves to cause atrial contraction. When atrial contraction occurs, the pressure in the chambers of the atria elevates. Increased atrial pressure forces increased blood flow across the AV valves. Increased blood flow across the AV valves results in rapid blood flow into the ventricles. About 10% of left ventricular filling is a result of atrial contraction while at rest.

Isovolumetric Contraction (Phase 2)

Phase 2 of the cardiac cycle originates with ventricular depolarization, which serves to cause excitation-contraction coupling, contraction of the myocytes, and a rapid elevation of intraventricular pressure. Maximal pressure development (max dP/dt) occurs early in this phase. When the intraventricular pressure becomes greater than the atrial pressure, the AV valves close. Between the closing of the AV valves and the opening of the aortic and pulmonic valves, the pressure in the ventricles elevates quickly with no change in volume. The volume in the ventricles does not change as all the valves are closed; thus, the contraction is termed isovolumetric.

Rapid Ejection (Phase 3)

Phase 3 of the cardiac cycle is when blood is initially and quickly ejected into the aorta and pulmonary arteries from the left and right ventricles. The increased intraventricular pressures are greater than the pressures in the aorta and pulmonary arteries, which function to open the aortic and pulmonic valves. The total energy of the blood in the ventricle is greater than the total energy of the blood in the aorta, which results in ejection of blood secondary to the presence of an energy gradient. During this phase, the ventricular pressure is greater than the outflow tract pressure.

Reduced Ejection (Phase 4)

Phase 4 of the cardiac cycle begins with ventricular repolarization, which happens about 200 msec after the QRS and the beginning of contraction of the ventricles. Ventricular repolarization results in a decrease in the active tension in the ventricles. The decrease in the active tension in the ventricles leads to a decrease in the ventricular emptying or the rate of ejection of the blood. The pressure in the ventricles decreases to less than the pressure of the outflow tract; however, the flow is still outward secondary to the kinetic (inertial) energy of the blood. The aortic and pulmonic valves are open, while the atrioventricular valves are closed.

Isovolumetric Relaxation (Phase 5)

Isovolumetric relaxation, or phase 5 of the cardiac cycle, begins with ventricular repolarization, which happens about 200 msec after the QRS begins with the closure of the aortic and pulmonic valves as a result of the decrease in the intraventricular pressures. The closure of the valves causes the dicrotic notch seen in the aortic and pulmonary artery pressure tracings. After the valves close, there is a slight increase in the pressure in the aorta and pulmonary arteries that is then followed by a slight decrease in pressure. The pressure in the ventricles decreases during this phase, but the volume stays constant, as all the valves remain closed.

Rapid Filling (Phase 6)

When the intraventricular pressures decline below the atrial pressures, the atrioventricular (AV) valves quickly open. Opening of the AV valves subsequently results in ventricular filling. As the ventricles are still relaxing early in this phase, the intraventricular pressures continue to decrease even though blood is flowing from the atria. With complete ventricular relaxation, the pressure in the ventricles elevates secondary to inflow of blood from the atria. When the mitral valve opens, a rapid decline in left atrial pressure results; similar events occur in the right atrial pressure with the opening of the tricuspid valve.

Describe Reduced Filling (Phase 7)

Reduced filling, or phase 7 of the cardiac cycle, is when the atrioventricular (AV) valves open. The ventricles become filled with blood and expand in size. At this point, the ventricles are less compliant, which results in elevation of the intraventricular pressures. The pressure gradient over the AV valves is decreased. A reduction in the pressure gradient across the AV valves causes the rate of filling to decline. Approximately 90% of the ventricle is filled with blood at the end of phase 7 in a normal heart at rest; therefore, 90% of ventricular filling happens prior to atrial contraction (phase 1).

Response to Exercise Stress Testing

Exercise stress testing is a means to test the cardiovascular response to stress by exercising on a treadmill or bicycle while the electrocardiogram (EKG) and blood pressure are monitored. Dynamic exercise results in elevations of ventricular heart rate, stroke volume, and cardiac output. Early in the exercising period, cardiac output is elevated by augmentation of the stroke volume by means of the Starling mechanism and heart rate. Later during the exercise, increased cardiac output is secondary to increased ventricular rate. The age-predicted maximum heart rate is used for safety measures and to provide a basis for the appropriate stress to cause ischemia. A value of 90% of age-predicted maximum heart rate is considered to be an excellent result.

Review Video: EKG Rhythms - Reading the Graph
Visit mometrix.com/academy and enter code: 872282

Response to Pharmacologic Stress Testing

A pharmacologic agent is used to create cardiac stress in patients unable to exercise or patients with decreased functional capacity. The typical agents for pharmacologic stress testing are adenosine, dipyridamole, and dobutamine, which are vasodilators that cause increased blood velocity and rate of flow in normal vessels and decreased response in abnormal vessels. A normal response does not demonstrate cardiac steal of flow or perfusion defects on nuclear cardiac scans or ST-segment changes on electrocardiography (EKG). Normal results at rest and after stress typically indicate normal coronary artery blood flow.

Timing of the Cardiac Cycle and EKG

The waveforms on the electrocardiogram (EKG) are divided into segments that serve to measure phases of the cardiac cycle. The repetitive aspect of the cardiac cycle is the "P-QRS-T" waveform. The P wave reflects atrial depolarization or contraction, which represents when the sinus rhythm beat electrically captures the left and right atria. The QRS complex reflects ventricular depolarization or contraction. The length of the QRS complex typifies ventricular disease. The PR interval is a measurement of the time it takes for atrial contraction to reach the ventricle. The QT interval reflects ventricular activity and recovery with the T wave reflecting the recovery phase.

Pericardium

The pericardium is a two-layered thin membrane that contains the heart and the roots of the great vessels. The pericardium has a vital role in protecting and stabilizing the heart. Another function of the pericardium is to provide lubrication for the heart's surface and to restrict cardiac enlargement. The pericardium also serves to anchor the heart via ligamentous attachments, which assures that the heart is in proper position in the thoracic cavity. The pericardium and its ligamentous attachments also serve to prevent the heart from moving and protect the organ from damage and infection.

Function of the Pericardium in the Regulation of Cardiovascular Hemodynamics

One of the functions of the pericardium is to curtail diastolic expansion that ultimately restrains the work of the ventricle when subjected to elevated atrial or end-diastolic ventricular pressures. If the left ventricle becomes overstressed and dilated, the pericardium functions to curtail the diastolic expansion of the right ventricle and thus limits the work of the right ventricle. By limiting the work of the right ventricle, the pulmonary capillary pressures and the left atrial pressures are also lowered. The pericardium also serves to protect against tricuspid and mitral regurgitation in the presence of elevated ventricular filling pressures.

Pleura

The pleura functions to surround the lungs and is comprised of two serous membranes: (1) the parietal pleura and (2) the visceral pleura. The outer layer is the parietal pleura, which serves to cover the lungs and attaches to the chest wall; the inner layer is the visceral pleura, which also covers the lungs and the blood vessels, bronchi, and nerves. There is a thin space in between the two layers of pleura that contains pleural fluid. Pleural fluid functions to lubricate the pleural surfaces and to provide appropriate surface tension to enable optimal alveoli inflation.

Timing of Events Relative to the Respirometer

It is important to realize that respiration and thus use of the respirometer will cause cyclic physiological alterations in cardiac hemodynamics. Normal variations will be noted in the right and left ventricular Doppler inflows and outflows as well as alterations in extracardiac flows. Inspiration results in a decrease in intrathoracic and intrapericardial pressures and thus augments right ventricular filling. During expiration, the intrathoracic and intrapericardial pressures increase, which serves to decrease the diastolic filling pressure in the right ventricle and increase the filling of the left ventricle. Expiration provides improved parasternal and apical views of the heart.

Pathology

Abnormal Coronary Artery Origination and Course

Dr. Paolo Angelini classifies abnormalities of coronary artery origination and course as follows: absent main trunk [split left coronary artery (LCA)]; abnormal location of coronary ostium within aortic root; abnormal location of coronary ostium outside normal coronary sinuses (examples include right posterior aortic sinus, ascending aorta, left ventricle, right ventricle, pulmonary artery variants, aortic arch, innominate artery, right carotid artery, internal mammary artery, bronchial artery, subclavian artery, and descending aorta); abnormalities of the intrinsic coronary anatomy (examples include congenital ostial stenosis or atresia, absent coronary artery, and coronary artery hypoplasia); and abnormalities of termination of the coronary artery.

Segmental Wall Motion Abnormalities

Segmental wall motion abnormalities are also known as regional wall motion abnormalities. Such abnormalities refer to abnormal motion of a wall segment of the heart. Decreased segmental heart wall motion is known as hypokinesia. Absent segmental heart wall motion is termed akinesia. Increased segmental heart wall motion is called hyperkinesia. Segmental wall motion abnormalities can also be demonstrated by paradoxical wall motion, such as the wall segment bulging outward during systole as opposed to moving inward. Such paradoxical segmental wall motion is referred to as dyskinesia. The regional segmental wall dysfunction indicates which coronary artery may be diseased.

Right Ventricle Abnormalities

The right ventricle is thin walled, and therefore it is quite sensitive to any change in pulmonary artery pressures. A change in right ventricle size may be secondary to volume or pressure overload and may result in right ventricular hypertrophy. An example of right ventricular hypertrophy includes rapid elevation in pulmonary artery pressure secondary to a pulmonary embolism, which will result in enlargement of the right ventricle. Enlargement of the right ventricle in this instance will result in dilation of the annulus of the tricuspid valve with subsequent tricuspid regurgitation. In the presence of multivessel coronary artery disease, the right ventricle shows long-axis motion dysfunction.

Ventricular Aneurysms

A defect found in the left or right ventricle of the heart that produces a transmural infarction is a ventricular aneurysm. Ventricular aneurysms may be true aneurysms or false aneurysms. The true ventricular aneurysm is comprised of damaged myocardial wall, while a false ventricular aneurysm is actually a rupture that has a containing boundary such as pericardium as opposed to myocardium. Ventricular aneurysms bulge outward while other segments contract and thus hamper ventricular contractile ability and function. False ventricular aneurysms reflect localized rupture of the myocardium, whereas pericardial adhesions serve to limit hemorrhage.

Diseases of the Great Vessels

Diseases of the great vessels include diseases of the aorta, superior vena cava, inferior vena cava, and pulmonary arteries. Problems with the aorta can include thoracic aneurysms, aortic dissections, coarctation of the aorta, and traumatic injury. Abnormalities of the superior vena cava may include congenital abnormalities such as a persistent left superior vena cava, a right superior vena cava, and superior vena cava syndrome (typically due to compression from metastatic disease). The inferior vena cava may exhibit inferior vena cava syndrome. Disease of the pulmonary artery may be a result of pulmonary hypertension or pulmonary artery stenosis.

Aortic Aneurysm

An aneurysm may present at any location in the aorta. It is characterized as a localized or diffuse dilation of an artery with a diameter that is at least 50% greater than normal artery size. Thoracic aorta aneurysms are classed into three groups based on location: ascending aorta, aortic arch, and descending thoracic or thoracoabdominal. Aneurysms of the ascending aorta may be located proximally to the annulus of the aorta or distally to the innominate artery. Descending aortic aneurysms typically originate at a location beyond the left subclavian artery.

Aortic Atheroma

An aortic atheroma is the result of the accumulation of lipid-rich plaque in the intima that also affects the structure and function of the media of the aorta. The pathophysiology of aortic atheroma is thought to be related to damage of the endothelium, which enables the deposition of low-density lipoproteins (LDLs) into the intima. Macrophages subsequently secrete cytokines that stimulate the proliferation of intimal cells. The intimal cells develop fibroblastic characteristics and secrete collagen. Collagen causes plaque fibrosis, which results in pressure atrophy of the aortic media and disruption of the elastic lamina. Aortic atheroma may result in decreased blood flow, predisposition to thrombosis, plaque hemorrhage, and vessel wall weakening with aneurysm formation.

Pathophysiology of Aortic Dissection

The wall of the aorta is subject to increased pulsatile pressure and shear stress that contribute to the aorta's vulnerability to injury and disease as a result of mechanical trauma. Aortic dissection is a horizontal or diagonal split in the media of the aorta. Aortic dissection presents with the appearance of a double-barreled aorta as a result of an intimal tear that links the media with the lumen of the aorta. An exit tear functions to establish a true lumen and a false lumen that cause the double-barreled appearance.

Anatomic Locations and Classifications of Aortic Dissection

Most aortic dissections originate in three classic anatomic locations. The most common anatomic locations are 2.2 cm above the root of the aorta, distal to the left subclavian artery, and the aortic arch. Ninety percent of dissections are located within 10 cm of the aortic valve; the second most common location is distal to the left subclavian artery. Dissection of the ascending aorta may result in death secondary to wall rupture, hemopericardium and tamponade, coronary ostial occlusion and myocardial infarction, or aortic insufficiency. The DeBakey classification of aortic dissection is as follows: type I (ascending and descending aorta), type II (ascending aorta only), and type III (descending aorta only).

Sinus of Valsalva Aneurysm

A sinus of Valsalva aneurysm is typically a rare congenital issue that may be clinically silent or cause compression of surrounding cardiac structures or intracardiac shunting as a result of rupture into the right heart. Approximately 65% to 85% of these aneurysms are located at the right sinus of Valsalva; noncoronary origins account for 10% to 30%; and origination in the left sinus of Valsalva accounts for less than 5%. Most sinus of Valsalva aneurysms are of congenital origin; however, other disease processes may also cause these aneurysms, such as atherosclerotic aneurysms, syphilis, endocarditis, cystic medial necrosis, and chest trauma.

Mitral Valve Stenosis

The narrowing of the inlet valve into the left ventricle that stops proper filling during diastole is known as mitral stenosis. The valve leaflets in mitral stenosis may be thickened, have commissural fusion, or have thick or short subvalvular structures. Causes of mitral stenosis are almost always secondary to rheumatic fever but may also be due to mucopolysaccharidoses, severe annular calcification, congenital abnormalities, disorders of serotonin metabolism, methysergide treatment, or systemic autoimmune disorders such as lupus or rheumatoid arthritis. The 10-year survival in untreated mitral stenosis is 50% to 60%, with congestive heart failure, systemic emboli, pulmonary embolism, and infection being the causes of death.

Mitral Annular Calcification

Mitral annular calcification is recurrent degenerative process of the mitral valve ring. Mitral annular calcification is typically considered to be the result of an inflammatory process. There is a strong link between mitral annular calcification and atherosclerosis; the mitral annulus is the site of turbulent blood flow that may induce endothelial damage and the subsequent deposition of lipids and associated inflammatory mediators. Mitral annular calcification is intensified and progresses more rapidly by advanced age, systemic hypertension, elevated cholesterol, diabetes, chronic renal failure and secondary hyperparathyroidism, Marfan syndrome, and Hurler syndrome.

Aortic Valve Stenosis

Stenosis of the aortic valve results in the obstruction of the flow of blood across the aortic valve. Aortic valve stenosis may be secondary to a congenital cause (unicuspid or bicuspid valve) or calcific degeneration, or it may be rheumatic in origin. The current leading indication for aortic valve replacement is calcific degeneration of the aortic valve. Acquired aortic valve stenosis has the following etiologies: hypertension, high cholesterol, diabetes, and smoking. Other causes include rheumatic heart disease, obstructive valve vegetations, homozygous type II hypercholesterolemia, Paget disease, Fabry disease, ochronosis, and irradiation. Rheumatic heart disease that involves the aortic valve often also involves the mitral valve.

Tricuspid Valve Stenosis

Tricuspid valve stenosis may be secondary to structural abnormalities of the valve or from functional abnormalities of the myocardium. Tricuspid stenosis is almost always a result of rheumatic heart disease and is usually associated with aortic and mitral valve issues. Tricuspid valve stenosis secondary to rheumatic fever presents with valve leaflets that appear thickened and sclerotic. Tricuspid valve stenosis results in obstruction of blood flow into the right ventricle and therefore into the pulmonary vessels. Tricuspid stenosis causes right atrial enlargement, hepatomegaly, diminished pulmonary blood flow, and peripheral edema. Other causes of tricuspid stenosis include carcinoid syndrome, endocarditis, endomyocardial fibrosis, lupus, and congenital tricuspid atresia.

Pulmonic Valve Stenosis

Pulmonic valve stenosis is usually congenital in origin, but it may rarely be secondary to carcinoid syndrome or rheumatic fever. The pulmonic valve may exhibit stenotic leaflets, atretic leaflets, or absent leaflets. The location of pulmonic stenosis may be valvar, supravalvar, subvalvar, or in the branch pulmonary arteries. Pulmonic valve stenosis usually presents with a valve that appears shaped like a dome secondary to the fusion of the leaflets of the valve. About 8% to 12% of congenital heart defects in children are due to pulmonic stenosis, while 15% of congenital heart defects in adults are due to pulmonic stenosis.

Pathophysiology of Mitral Valve Regurgitation

Mitral valve regurgitation is typically a result of rheumatic fever or mitral valve prolapse; mitral valve prolapse is the most common cause in the Western world (45%). Mitral regurgitation is usually classified in three stages. The three stages are acute, chronic compensated, and chronic decompensated. Acute mitral valve regurgitation is most commonly a result of a myocardial infarction with spontaneous rupture of the chordae tendineae or the papillary muscle. After the acute stage, chronic compensation results; eccentric left ventricular hypertrophy and left ventricular dysfunction then develop. Chronic decompensation results in increased left atrial pressure and subsequent congestion of the pulmonary system.

Rupture of the Chordae Tendineae or the Papillary Muscle

Normal mitral valve function is a result of the interaction between the annulus of the mitral valve, leaflets, chordae, papillary muscle, and the myocardium of the left ventricle. A ruptured papillary muscle is a rare cause of mitral regurgitation and occurs in about 1% of acute myocardial infarctions. The most commonly ruptured papillary muscle is the posteromedial papillary muscle. Papillary muscles are vulnerable to ischemia secondary to a limited blood supply and an elevated oxygen demand; ischemia thus results in rupture and fibrosis. Alteration in the anatomy after rupture distorts the leaflets of the valve and leads to regurgitation.

Flail Leaflet

A flail leaflet is the result of a ruptured chordae tendineae and is the most likely reason in Western society for surgical repair of mitral regurgitation. A flail leaflet secondary to rupture of the chordae may be due to congenital abnormality, spontaneous primary rupture, infective endocarditis, trauma, osteogenesis imperfecta, relapsing polychondritis, acute dilation of the left ventricle, and increased mechanical strain. Flail leaflets are more common in males and in younger patients; therefore, early surgical correction is usually undertaken. There is a higher incidence of death, congestive heart failure, thromboembolism, atrial fibrillation, hemorrhage, and endocarditis with flail leaflets.

Mitral Valve Prolapse

Mitral valve prolapse may be noted in numerous disorders and typically is a normal variant as opposed to an isolated disease entity. Mitral valve prolapse increases the risk of arrhythmias, endocarditis, cerebrovascular accident, mitral regurgitation, mitral valve replacement, and sudden death. The pathophysiology of mitral valve prolapse is usually secondary to myxomatous degeneration from collagen dissolution in the middle spongiosa layer of the mitral valve leaflets. This results in lengthening of the leaflets and the chordae tendineae. Cardiac aspects of mitral valve prolapse include supraventricular arrhythmias, palpitations, mitral regurgitation, sudden death, and cerebral ischemia.

Aortic Valve Regurgitation

Aortic valve regurgitation is the backward flow of blood across the aortic valve that occurs during diastole. Aortic valve regurgitation causes a volume overload in the left ventricle. Acute aortic regurgitation does not result in changes to the left ventricle, whereas chronic aortic regurgitation results in enlargement and eccentric hypertrophy of the left ventricle. Acute aortic regurgitation results in acute volume overload in the left ventricle that subsequently increases the pulmonary venous pressure. This elevated pulmonary venous pressure may cause dyspnea, pulmonary edema, and congestive heart failure, and it may even deteriorate into cardiogenic shock.

Chronic Aortic Valve Regurgitation

Chronic aortic valve regurgitation results in a gradual increase in left ventricular volume overload that results in left ventricular enlargement and eccentric left ventricular hypertrophy. When the left ventricle enlarges, it becomes more compliant and thus produces a greater stroke volume to compensate for the larger volume load. The ejection fraction is normal or elevated in the early aspects of chronic aortic regurgitation; however, as the left ventricular pressure becomes greater than the preload reserves, the ejection fraction decreases. Once the left ventricle reaches maximum diameter, the diastolic pressures elevate, which results in symptoms.

Etiologies of Aortic Valve Regurgitation

Aortic valve regurgitation may be secondary to valvular disease or aortic root disease. Abnormalities of the aortic valve that may result in regurgitation include bicuspid aortic valve (the most common congenital etiology), rheumatic fever, infective endocarditis, collagen vascular diseases, and degenerative disease of the aortic valve. Diseases of the ascending aorta may also cause aortic valve regurgitation and include chronic uncontrolled hypertension, Marfan syndrome, idiopathic dilation of the aorta, cystic medial necrosis, senile aortic ectasia and dilation, syphilitic aortitis, giant cell arteritis, Takayasu arteritis, ankylosing spondylitis, Whipple disease, and various other forms of spondyloarthropathy.

Tricuspid Valve Regurgitation

If abnormalities of the tricuspid valve exist, regurgitation may result. Abnormalities may involve the leaflets of the valve, the chordae tendineae, annulus of the valve, papillary muscles, or the adjacent right ventricle. An incompetent tricuspid valve may be due to primary defects of the leaflets or the chordae or due to secondary issues with myocardial function and dilation. Endocarditis or rheumatic fever may cause tricuspid regurgitation. Rheumatic fever commonly results in both tricuspid regurgitation and stenosis. The most frequent congenital cause of tricuspid regurgitation is Ebstein anomaly. Tricuspid regurgitation results in right ventricular volume overload and right heart failure with subsequent hepatic congestion, peripheral edema, and ascites.

Pulmonic Valve Regurgitation

Pulmonic valve regurgitation is the backward flow of blood across the pulmonic valve. The backward blood flow is from the pulmonary artery into the right ventricle during diastole. Almost all people have physiologic (trace-to-mild) pulmonic regurgitation. Clinically significant pulmonic valve regurgitation results in abnormal right ventricle function and right-sided heart failure. Pulmonic valve regurgitation is typically a result of an underlying disease process such as pulmonary hypertension or dilated cardiomyopathy. Pulmonic valve regurgitation is caused by an incompetent pulmonic valve secondary to dilation of the pulmonic valve ring, acquired structural defects of the leaflets, or congenital malformations.

Identifying Tricuspid Prolapse on Echo

Isolated tricuspid prolapse is rare; tricuspid prolapse usually occurs in conjunction with mitral valve prolapse. The echocardiographic patterns of tricuspid prolapse are similar in appearance to those of mitral valve prolapse. The tricuspid valve echo shows either midsystolic posterior motion or hammock-like posterior motion that begins in early systole. During systole, the normal tricuspid valve pattern is that of gradual anterior movement. Midsystolic motion characterizing tricuspid prolapse shows initial horizontal movement that is then followed by posterior valve movement. Hammock-like posterior motion shows early systolic posterior motion with anterior motion in the latter portion of systole.

Abnormalities of the Coronary Sinus

Typically, the coronary sinus opens into the right atrium and is responsible for 75% of the venous circulation of the heart by means of blood return from most of the regions of the heart. Dr. Emil Mantini classified coronary sinus abnormalities as enlargement of the coronary sinuses with/without left-to-right shunt, absent coronary sinus, atresia of the right atrial coronary sinus ostium, and hypoplasia of the coronary sinus. An enlarged coronary sinus is often associated with abnormal systemic venous return or a left-to-right shunt. An absent coronary sinus is very rare and is always linked to a persistent left superior vena cava connection to the left atrium and atrial septal defect.

Pericardial Abnormalities

Pericardial abnormalities include acute pericarditis, constrictive pericarditis, pericardial effusion, and cardiac tamponade. Acute pericarditis is an inflammation of the pericardium that may be primary or secondary to systemic disease. Causes may include infection (viral, bacterial, or fungal); autoimmune disorders [systemic lupus erythematous (SLE), rheumatoid arthritis (RA)]; medications (hydralazine, procainamide); Dressler's syndrome; in the first five days post transmural myocardial infarction; malignancy; postoperative cardiac surgery; trauma; radiation; uremia; or myxedema. Constrictive pericarditis causes the heart to be enclosed in a rigid pericardium and may be idiopathic, secondary to tuberculosis (TB), or as a result of acute pericarditis. A pericardial effusion may be secondary to any form of acute pericarditis.

Aortic Arch Abnormalities

The five primary types of aortic arch abnormalities are as follows: (1) double aortic arch, (2) right aortic arch with normal branching, (3) right aortic arch with abnormal branching, (4) left aortic arch with abnormal branching, and (5) cervical aortic arch. Aortic arch abnormalities may also be classified into those that result in physiologic abnormalities and those that do not result in physiologic abnormalities. Physiologic abnormalities that are a result of aortic arch anomalies include tracheobronchial compression, esophageal compression, and abnormal patterns of blood flow. Tracheobronchial and esophageal compression are typically secondary to a vascular ring from a double aortic arch.

Abnormalities of the Hepatic Veins

Normally, the three main hepatic veins in most adults are the right, middle, and left hepatic veins; the middle and left veins join just before their entry into the inferior vena cava. Budd–Chiari syndrome is a rare disorder caused by occlusion of the hepatic veins. The occlusion of the hepatic veins may be located at any level. When occlusion of the hepatic venules occurs post bone marrow transplant, the condition is known as hepatic veno-occlusive disease. Occlusion of the hepatic veins yields a classic triad of hepatomegaly, ascites, and abdominal pain.

Causes of Prosthetic Valve Dysfunction

Prosthetic valve dysfunction may be secondary to structural deterioration, paravalvular regurgitation, patient–prosthetic mismatch, thrombosis, and endocarditis. Structural deterioration may be a result of valve wear, leaflet tear, leaflet fracture, calcification, and suture line disruption. Structural deterioration typically presents as prosthetic valve stenosis or regurgitation. Calcium deposition is a primary cause of structural prosthetic valve dysfunction because calcium deposition inhibits leaflet motion and initiates tears in the leaflets. Paravalvular leak is typically a result of endocarditis but may be secondary to poor positioning of the valve. Patient–prosthetic mismatch is due to an improperly sized valve.

Prosthetic Heart Valves

Prosthetic heart valves are either mechanical or bioprosthetic (also known as tissue valves). Some examples of single tilting-disc mechanical valves are as follows: Björk–Shiley (discontinued), Medtronic–Hall, Monostrut, OmniScience, Omnicarbon, and Lillehei–Kaster, and Ultracor (not available in the United States). Examples of bileaflet tilting-disc mechanical valves are St. Jude Medical, Carbomedics, Duromedics (discontinued), and ATS Medical Open Pivot (investigational). Nontilting disc mechanical valves have been discontinued but include Kay–Suzuki, Kay–Shiley, and Beall. Ball-in-cage mechanical valves include the Starr–Edwards. Heterograft bioprosthetic grafts are porcine-stented (Hancock, Carpentier–Edwards, Biocor, Epic, Intact, Mosaic); porcine unstented (St. Jude Toronto SPV, Medtronic Freestyle, Baxter Prima, CryoLife–O'Brien, Biocor); or bovine pericardial (Ionescu–Shiley, Hancock, Carpentier–Edwards Perimount, Mitroflow). Homografts and pulmonary autografts may also be used as valves.

Heart Valve Repairs

Heart valve repairs often may be accomplished without the use of artificial materials. The advantages of heart valve repairs include decreased risk of infection, decreased need for anticoagulants, and preservation of cardiac muscle strength. The mitral valve is the most common valve to be repaired. Commissurotomy is a type of heart valve repair in which fused leaflets are separated in order to establish a wider valve opening. Decalcification involves removing calcium deposits from valve leaflets. Triangular resection entails removing a floppy segment and suturing the remaining aspects together. Annuloplasty involves reshaping or tightening the annulus of the valve.

Ischemic Heart Disease

Ischemic heart disease is also known as coronary artery disease. Complications secondary to ischemic heart disease may include cardiac arrhythmias such as ventricular tachycardia, heart block, atrial fibrillation, and sudden death; congestive heart failure; Dressler's syndrome; myocardial infarction; mitral regurgitation; pericarditis; pulmonary embolism; shock; cerebrovascular accident; and ventricular aneurysm. Dressler's syndrome, which may develop after a myocardial infarction, is thought to be an autoimmune response involving the pericardium with resultant pericarditis. Mitral regurgitation may follow a myocardial infarction and then lead to the development of congestive heart failure. A ventricular aneurysm may occur after a large myocardial infarction.

True Aneurysms and Pseudoaneurysms

A ventricular aneurysm is a complication of myocardial infarction. True aneurysms cause a thin myocardium that is dyskinetic and includes all of the wall. A rupture of the ventricular free wall may result in a pseudoaneurysm, which is contained by the overlying pericardium. A pseudoaneurysm usually has a narrower neck than the aneurysmal diameter and occurs in the posterior or lateral wall. True aneurysms typically have a wider neck and occur in the anterior wall or apex. A pseudoaneurysm has a greater risk of rupture.

Ischemic Ventricular Septal Defect

An ischemic ventricular septal defect typically is the result of a myocardial infarction and is defined as a rupture of the interventricular septum. It is quite rare but very serious because it can lead to myocardial rupture. Anterior ventricular septal rupture is due to an anterolateral myocardial infarction. An inferoseptal myocardial infarction may result in a posterior ventricular septal rupture. The ischemic ventricular septal defect typically occurs two or three days post myocardial infarction; 85% of these patients will die in two months if surgical repair is not accomplished. Medical treatment without surgery results in a mortality rate of over 90%.

Dilated Cardiomyopathy

Dilated cardiomyopathy presents with enlargement of the chambers of the ventricle and systolic dysfunction. The left ventricle is enlarged, but little to no ventricular hypertrophy is exhibited. The impairment of the systolic function results in elevated end-diastolic and end-systolic volumes. Progression of dilated cardiomyopathy may result in significant mitral and tricuspid regurgitation. Subsequent mitral and tricuspid regurgitation results in decreased cardiac output, elevated end-systolic volumes, and increased stress on the wall of the ventricle. There are multiple causes of dilated cardiomyopathy; some examples include genetics, ischemic heart disease, infection, metabolic disorders, nutrition, and toxins.

Isolated Left Ventricular Noncompaction

Isolated left ventricular noncompaction is extremely rare and has been categorized as a primary genetic cardiomyopathy by the American Heart Association. Left ventricular noncompaction has the following elements, according to Dobranici *et al.* in the *Journal of Medicine and Life* (2012; **5**: 110–113): "(1) altered myocardial wall with prominent trabeculae and deep intertrabecular recesses resulting in thickened myocardium with two layers consisting of compacted and noncompacted myocardium and (2) continuity between the left ventricular cavity and the deep intertrabecular recesses, which are filled with blood from the ventricular cavity without evidence of communication to the pericardial coronary system." Complications of left ventricular noncompaction may include decreased systolic function, ventricular arrhythmias, and systemic embolization.

Hypertrophic Cardiomyopathy

Hypertrophic cardiomyopathy is an autosomal-dominant condition that has variable penetrance and variable expressivity. It is the leading reason for sudden cardiac death in preadolescents and adolescents. The classic feature of hypertrophic cardiomyopathy is asymmetric myocardial hypertrophy that is not the result of an inciting stimulus for hypertrophy. The hypertrophy may be demonstrated in any area of the left ventricle but is most often noted in the interventricular septum and causes flow obstruction in the left ventricular outflow tract. Some cases do not cause obstruction but still pose a great risk of sudden cardiac death secondary to arrhythmia.

Asymmetrical Septal Hypertrophy

Asymmetrical septal hypertrophy may occur with or without obstruction. The most common form is without obstruction in which the hypertrophy is present primarily in the center of the septum and does not result in obstruction of blood flow from the left ventricular outflow tract. Asymmetrical septal hypertrophy without obstruction also does not involve the mitral valve, which is in the normal position. Asymmetrical hypertrophy with obstruction results in blood flow obstruction from the left ventricular outflow tract because the narrowing of the outflow tract from the hypertrophy allows the mitral valve to press against the septum.

Systolic Anterior Motion of the Mitral Valve

Systolic anterior motion of the mitral valve is described as an anterior and posterior paradoxical motion of the mitral valve leaflet moving to the left ventricular outflow tract during systole. The mechanism of systolic anterior motion of the mitral valve has been postulated to be secondary to a Venturi effect or to anatomic positional abnormalities of the papillary muscles and the leaflets of the mitral valve. Systolic anterior motion of the mitral valve is most commonly found in asymmetrical septal hypertrophy but may also be found in hypertensive heart disease, diabetes, acute myocardial infarction (MI), and after mitral valve repair. A characteristic noted on echocardiography is midsystolic notching of the aortic valve.

Restrictive Cardiomyopathy

Restrictive cardiomyopathy is a rare disorder of the myocardium, defined by the World Health Organization as "a myocardial disease characterized by restrictive filling and reduced diastolic volume of either or both ventricles with normal or near-normal systolic function and wall thickness." Restrictive cardiomyopathy may be idiopathic or may be secondary to disease of the myocardium, such as amyloidosis. This disorder has four categories: (1) idiopathic, (2) infiltrative, (3) treatment induced, and (4) malignant. Patients will present with congestive heart failure and dynamics that are consistent with restriction but will not exhibit significant ventricular hypertrophy or endocardial fibrosis.

Two-Dimensional Echocardiogram (2D Echo) Findings with Restrictive Cardiomyopathy

It is critical to correctly distinguish between constrictive pericarditis and restrictive cardiomyopathy because the treatment approaches are vastly different. On 2D echo, restrictive cardiomyopathy demonstrates a left ventricle that is not dilated, not hypertrophied, and contracts in a normal manner. Both atria exhibit profound dilation. The size of the cavity of the ventricle will be either normal or decreased. The thickness of the ventricular wall may be greater than normal in cases of infiltrative disease such as amyloidosis. Infiltrative disease may also demonstrate abnormal texture of the myocardium.

Hypertensive Heart Disease

Hypertensive heart disease is the result of long-standing elevated blood pressure. Chronic and poorly controlled hypertension results in numerous alterations in the structure of the myocardium, coronary vessels, and the electrical conduction system. Such alterations often lead to left ventricular hypertrophy, coronary artery disease, disorders of the conduction system, and systolic and diastolic abnormalities. Complications secondary to hypertensive heart disease and changes in the heart include angina, myocardial infarction, arrhythmias (especially atrial fibrillation), and congestive heart failure. Approximately 15% to 20% of patients with hypertensive heart disease will demonstrate left ventricular hypertrophy and structural changes in the left atrium.

The echocardiogram is a noninvasive procedure of choice in the evaluation of the effects of hypertensive heart disease. Hypertension is one of the more common causes of left ventricular hypertrophy as well as congestive heart failure. Echocardiography may be used to evaluate left ventricular hypertrophy and the function of the left ventricle in patients with systemic hypertension. Concentric remodeling of the left ventricle is frequently seen in hypertensive heart disease. Diastolic filling abnormalities may also be noted with or without systolic abnormalities in hypertensive heart disease. Left ventricular compliance may also be measured.

Pulmonary Hypertension

Pulmonary hypertension may be primary or secondary; primary pulmonary hypertension does not have an underlying cause. Secondary pulmonary hypertension may be due to chronic pulmonary disease such as cystic fibrosis, chronic obstructive pulmonary disease, or obstructive sleep apnea; recurrent thrombosis; congestive heart failure; rheumatologic disease such as rheumatoid arthritis (RA), systemic lupus erythematosus (SLE), or scleroderma; street drug use such as cocaine, speed, or methamphetamine; weight-loss drugs such as Fen-Phen; HIV; AIDS; hyperthyroidism; and advanced hepatic disease. Pulmonary hypertension is defined by Dr. Richard Klabunde (http://www.cvpharmacology.com/clinical%20topics/pulmonary%20hypertension-2.htm) as "a mean pulmonary arterial pressure greater than 25 mmHg at rest or greater than 30 mm HG during exercise."

Pulmonary hypertension ultimately results in pressure overload of the right heart. Some M-mode findings of pulmonary hypertension include an absent or decreased "a" dip of < 2mm of the cusps of the pulmonary valves, which is indicative of elevated pulmonary artery end-diastolic pressure, and the "flying W" that indicates midsystolic notching of the cusp of the pulmonary valve. Dilation of the right ventricle is an early finding in pulmonary hypertension and occurs in the short axis. Tricuspid and pulmonary regurgitation follow right ventricular dilation; right atrial dilation is a late result of pulmonary hypertension.

Detection of Coronary Artery Disease

During Exercise Stress Testing

Exercise stress testing has been used to detect the risk of coronary artery disease for more than 60 years. Abnormalities during exercise stress testing may include abnormal ST-segment response [horizontal, planar, or downsloping of >1 mm (0.5 mm or 2 mm are sometimes used as cut-off points)]; T-wave elevation of >1 mm in leads without Q waves; and T-wave changes such as inversion and pseudonormalization (when an inverted T wave becomes upright). There are specific criteria for discontinuing a test, which include electrocardiography (EKG) and clinical findings.

Using Pharmacologic Stress Testing

An abnormal result of a pharmacologic stress test is generally thought to be a reversible perfusion abnormality. Some centers, however, consider a fixed perfusion defect, especially without a history of previous myocardial infarction, to be a positive result. Pharmacologic stress testing can identify a stenotic coronary artery by highlighting abnormalities in the myocardial areas supplied by the coronary artery. The extent of coronary artery disease may also be ascertained by assessing the number of locations with perfusion abnormalities or defects. Pharmacologic stress testing is preferred in patients with a left bundle branch block.

Abnormal Physiology of Diastolic Dysfunction

Diastolic dysfunction is described as changes in ventricular diastolic properties that have a negative effect on stroke volume. End-diastolic volume or ventricular filling depends on venous return and ventricular compliance in diastole. Decreased ventricular compliance causes decreased ventricular filling and elevated end-diastolic pressure; this serves to decrease the stroke volume. A decrease in the stroke volume also causes a decrease in ventricular stroke work. Left ventricular involvement in diastolic dysfunction results in elevated pressures in the left atrium and the pulmonary venous pressures, which results in pulmonary edema. Right ventricular involvement results in elevated pressures in the right atrium and systemic venous system, which results in peripheral edema and ascites.

Physiology of Systolic Dysfunction

Systolic dysfunction is described by ventricular contraction that is impaired from the changes in signal transduction mechanisms that regulate inotropy or from the loss of viable, contracting muscle. Systolic dysfunction causes elevation in ventricular end-diastolic pressure, which functions as a compensatory mechanism secondary to the Frank–Starling means to increase stroke volume. Changes also occur in systemic vascular resistance, blood volume, and venous pressures. The sympathetic nervous system serves to increase systemic vascular resistance and also increase venous pressure.

Sinus Node Disease

Normal sinus rhythm is usually a result of rapid spontaneous depolarization in the sinus node. The sinus node may become diseased and therefore lose the ability for spontaneous depolarization or the ability to mount an adequate response to autonomic stimulation. Sinus node disease may be exhibited by a decrease in the rate or even a complete cessation of the rate. Electrocardiographic (EKG) findings of sinus node disease include sinus bradycardia, sinus pauses, prolonged sinus arrest, and transient asystole. The atrioventricular (AV) node may then take over because it is the next fastest region of spontaneous depolarization and exhibits a nodal rhythm on EKG.

First-Degree Atrioventricular (AV) Block

Damage to the atrioventricular (AV) node often results in AV block. A first-degree AV block is the least serious form of AV block, wherein the AV node exhibits a decreased rate of conduction without failure of conduction. Normally, there is a slight delay of electrical depolarization traveling from the atria to the AV node; this is the PR interval on the EKG. A first-degree AV block demonstrates a longer delay than normally is seen in the AV node. The EKG will show a prolongation of the PR interval; the hallmark is >200 ms.

Second-Degree Atrioventricular (AV) Block

Progression of atrioventricular (AV) node disease may result in further delay in the AV node conduction and may also result in complete conduction failure. The least severe form of second-degree block is the Mobitz I or Wenckebach AV block. EKG findings of Mobitz I AV block are at slowly increasing PR intervals with each successive heartbeat. This continues until one P wave does not conduct to the ventricles. Then, the AV node conduction recovers and the process starts over. Mobitz II AV block is a more severe form and is characterized on EKG by conduction failure without prolongation of the PR interval.

Third-Degree Atrioventricular (AV) Block

The most serious form of atrioventricular (AV) block is third-degree AV block. Third-degree AV block is also known as complete AV block, and it is the result of complete conduction failure from the atria to the ventricles. The location of the block may be in the AV node itself or in more distal conduction sites. Electrocardiography (EKG) will demonstrate a total lack of a compatible relationship between P waves and QRS complexes. Ventricular asystole is usually prevented by a cardiac safety mechanism known as an escape rhythm, wherein the AV node spontaneously depolarizes and causes ventricular contraction.

Regional Wall Abnormalities with Coronary Territory

It is important to ascertain the coronary artery territory and areas of perfusion. The left main coronary artery supplies the whole left ventricle and most of the left atrium barring the posterior aspect of the interventricular septum if the posterior descending artery is from the right coronary artery. The left anterior descending artery supplies the front two-thirds of the interventricular septum, the front of the left ventricle, and the entire apex. The left circumflex artery supplies the obtuse heart margin and the whole posterior wall, the left atrium, and the back of the interventricular septum if the posterior descending artery originates from the circumflex artery.

Seven segments are demonstrated on the apical four-chamber view. The seven segments are as follows: (1) apex, (2) apical lateral, (3) apical septal, (4) midseptal, (5) midlateral, (6) basal septal, and (7) basal lateral. The left anterior descending artery or the left circumflex coronary artery may supply the apical segment. The left anterior descending artery supplies the apical septal and midseptal segments. The right coronary artery supplies the basal septal segment, and the left circumflex supplies the apical lateral, midlateral, and basal lateral segments. The apical two-chamber view demonstrates seven segments: (1) basal inferior and (2) midinferior (right coronary artery); (3) apical inferior, (4) basal anterior, and (5) midanterior (left anterior descending artery); and apical anterior [either (6) right coronary artery (RCA) or (7) left anterior descending (LAD)].

The parasternal short-axis view is typically done at three levels for the assessment of wall motion scores: (1) mitral valve level (demonstrates six segments), (2) papillary muscle level (demonstrates six segments), and the (3) apical level (demonstrates four segments). Apical level segments are apical septal, apical anterior, apical lateral, and apical inferior. Papillary muscle segments are midseptal, midanteroseptal, midanterior, midlateral, midposterior, and midinferior. Mitral valve level segments are basal septal, basal anteroseptal, basal anterior, basal lateral, basal posterior, and basal inferior (midinferior = RCA, midposterior = RCA/LCX, midseptal and midanteroseptal = LAD; midanterior = LAD/LCX, and midlateral = LCX).

Endocarditis

Infective endocarditis is an infection that involves one or more valves, the mural endocardium, or a septal defect that is found on the endocardial surface of the heart. Endocarditis is typically the result of nonbacterial thrombotic endocarditis, which is a consequence of turbulence or trauma to the endothelial surface of the heart. Endocarditis is typically characterized into three forms: (1) native valve endocarditis (NVE), acute and subacute, (2) prosthetic valve endocarditis (PVE), early and late, and (3) intravenous (IV) drug abuse endocarditis. Other types are pacemaker infectious endocarditis and nosocomial infectious endocarditis (NIE).

Echocardiography Findings of Endocarditis

Echocardiography is especially helpful in the diagnosis of endocarditis inpatients that clinically present with endocarditis but have nonspecific blood cultures. Visible vegetations are typically suggestive of a poorer prognosis. Sensitivity is 90% to 100% in patients demonstrating vegetations in native valve endocarditis and greater than 90% in those demonstrating vegetations in prosthetic valve endocarditis. In the case of pacemaker infective endocarditis, transesophageal echocardiography will demonstrate vegetations on the pacemaker leads or on the tricuspid valve in greater than 90% of patients. Echocardiography may also be used to predict the risk of systemic embolization and to detect abscesses.

Complications of Endocarditis

Complications of endocarditis may include myocardial infarction, pericarditis, arrhythmias, cardiac valve insufficiency, congestive heart failure, sinus of Valsalva aneurysm, abscess of the aortic root, abscess of the myocardium, arterial emboli, arterial infarction, mycotic aneurysms, arthritis, myositis, glomerulonephritis, acute renal failure, stroke syndromes, mesenteric abscess or infarction, and splenic abscess or infarction. Congestive heart failure secondary to aortic insufficiency is the most typical complication of subacute endocarditis, followed by arterial embolization (occurring in both acute and subacute endocarditis). The most likely areas for embolization are the coronary arteries, kidneys, brain, and the spleen.

Pericardial Effusion

The descending thoracic aorta is the landmark used to differentiate pleural effusion from pericardial effusion. Effusions that are located anterior to the descending thoracic aorta are pericardial, while those located posterior to the descending thoracic aorta are pleural effusions. An abnormal amount of and/or an abnormal character to fluid in the pericardium is known as pericardial effusion. The etiology of a pericardial effusion may be local, systemic, and unknown. Clinical symptoms of a pericardial effusion are typically secondary to the rate at which the fluid accumulates. For example, a rapid accumulation of as little as 80 cc of fluid may cause symptoms, wherein a slow accumulation of up to 2 liters may not cause symptoms.

Hemodynamic Consequences of Pericardial Effusion and/or Cardiac Tamponade

Slow or quick compression of the heart that is due to the accumulation of fluid, pus, blood, clots, or gas, as a result of effusion, trauma, or rupture of the heart in the pericardium is a life-threatening condition known as cardiac tamponade. A large pericardial effusion or cardiac tamponade initially results in increased intrapericardial pressure with resultant cardiac chamber compression. In essence, the heart has to compete with the greater pericardial volume for the static intrapericardial volume. Increased cardiac chamber compression results in decreased diastolic myocardial compliance and thus decreases inflow to the heart. The ultimate result is profound hypotension or cardiogenic shock.

Hemodynamic Consequences of Constrictive Pericarditis

Constrictive pericarditis is often secondary to the deposition of fibrin, which causes a pericardial effusion and subsequent chronic fibrotic scarring and calcification. The pericardium is comprised of two layers: the visceral and the parietal pericardium. In constrictive pericarditis, the two layers fuse as a result of inflammation and thickening. When this occurs, the potential space in between the two layers is lost; the ventricle will then cease to have distensibility. The lack of distensibility of the ventricle limits venous return to the heart, decreases ventricular filling, and results in the inability to have appropriate preload.

Constrictive and Restrictive Physiology

It is vital to differentiate between constrictive and restrictive physiology because the treatments are vastly different. Restrictive physiology is characterized by a large reduction in ventricular compliance that results in significant diastolic dysfunction but normal systolic function. The causes of restrictive cardiac disease include cardiac amyloidosis, cardiac sarcoidosis, hemochromatosis, scleroderma, metastatic disease, Loeffler syndrome, certain medications, Anderson–Fabry disease, glycogen storage disease, and idiopathic. Constrictive physiology is characterized by a normal myocardium that cannot distend secondary to the constriction of the pericardium. Respiratory variability is greater in constrictive disease than in restrictive disease.

Complications of Dilated Cardiomyopathy

Dilated cardiomyopathy causes the chambers of the heart to dilate, which, in turn, weakens the cardiac muscle. The dilation of the chambers of the heart decreases the inflow and outflow from the heart. The left ventricle is typically involved in dilated cardiomyopathy, but the right ventricle may also be affected. As progressive enlargement of either the left or right ventricle occurs, signs and symptoms of congestive heart failure present. About 50% of cases of dilated cardiomyopathy are idiopathic in nature. Complications of dilated cardiomyopathy include cardiac arrhythmias, blood clots, peripheral edema, and congestive heart failure.

Hemodynamic Consequences of Hypertrophic Cardiomyopathy

The abnormal cellular structure and the thickened cardiac muscle demonstrated in hypertrophic cardiomyopathy result in disruption of the electrical system, which causes cardiac arrhythmias. Some of the typical arrhythmias noted in hypertrophic cardiomyopathy include atrial fibrillation, ventricular tachycardia, and ventricular fibrillation. Hypertrophic cardiomyopathy may also result in outflow obstruction of blood from the heart with the symptoms of dyspnea on exertion, syncope, and chest pain. Hypertrophy of the myocardium may cause more rapid and forceful blood flow through the mitral valve and subsequent mitral regurgitation. The thickened myocardium also leads to decreased ventricular compliance and congestive heart failure.

Metastatic Cardiac Tumors

Metastatic cardiac tumors may mimic valvular heart disease and result in congestive heart failure. They can cause supraventricular and ventricular arrhythmias, defects in electrical conduction, syncope, embolism, and pericardial effusion. Most metastatic cardiac tumors occur in those patients with disseminated metastatic disease; a single metastasis to the heart is very rare. Studies demonstrate that 25% of patients who die from metastatic disease have cardiac metastases. The most likely origins of cardiac metastases are the following: lung carcinoma, breast carcinoma, esophageal carcinoma, lymphoma, leukemia, and malignant melanoma. Metastatic cardiac tumors are typically numerous and small.

Primary Cardiac Tumors

Primary cardiac tumors are extremely rare, and the most common is atrial myxoma (40% to 50%). Primary cardiac tumors typically cause symptoms as a result of a mass effect, tumor invasion, embolization, or from systemic metastases. Symptoms can be secondary to obstruction of blood flow, impaired valve function, or as a result of embolization. Primary cardiac tumors may cause syncope, angina, shortness of breath, peripheral edema, ascites, cardiogenic shock, cardiomyopathy, and pulmonary hypertension. The origin of a primary cardiac tumor may be the endocardium, the valves, residual primitive tissue rests, and the conduction system.

Ebstein's Anomaly

Ebstein's anomaly is a congenital malformation of the heart that features apical displacement of the septal and posterior tricuspid valve leaflets causing the atrialization of the right ventricle with a range of degrees of malformation and displacement of the anterior leaflet. Ebstein's anomaly is often accompanied by other forms of congenital, structural, and conduction system abnormalities such as intracardiac shunts, lesions of the valves, and accessory conduction pathways. The abnormal tricuspid valve leaflets result in tricuspid regurgitation, while atrialization of the right ventricle results in improper contraction and subsequent stagnation of blood in the right atrium.

Patent Ductus Arteriosus

Patent ductus arteriosus is one of the most typical congenital heart defects. It demonstrates continuous communication of the descending thoracic aorta and the pulmonary artery. This results in failure of the closure of the fetal ductus. Patent ductus arteriosus is typically diagnosed in infancy but can occasionally be diagnosed in adulthood. In the case of isolated patent ductus arteriosus, a left-to-right shunt is present. The magnitude of the open communication and pulmonary vascular resistance will determine the volume of the left-to-right shunt. The most common patent ductus arteriosus is a left aortic root remnant.

Tetralogy of Fallot

Tetraology of Fallot is a very common congenital heart defect. It is a cyanotic disorder because a right-to-left shunt exists in which there is a lack of blood flow to the lungs for oxygenation. There are four common aspects of tetralogy of Fallot:

right ventricular outflow obstruction, ventricular septal defect, dextroposition of the aorta, and right ventricular hypertrophy. The pathophysiology of tetralogy of Fallot is secondary to the lack of proper development of the right ventricular infundibulum, which causes improper alignment of the infundibular septum in an anterior-leftward direction with resultant right ventricular outflow obstruction.

Atrial Septal Defects

Atrial septal defects are one of the most typical congenital cardiac defects that may be recognized in an adult. An atrial septal defect is a defect of the interatrial septum that allows the pulmonary venous return from the left atrium to go into the right atrium. The extent of the defect, shunting, and the presence of other abnormalities determine the extent of the disease. Symptoms may range from none to right-sided volume overload, pulmonary artery hypertension, and atrial arrhythmias. More than 70% of atrial septal defects are diagnosed in adults in their fifth decade.

Coarctation of the Aorta

Approximately 5% to 8% of all congenital cardiac defects are secondary to coarctation of the aorta. Coarctation of the aorta may be a solitary issue, or it may be associated with bicuspid aortic valve and ventricular septal defect or other cardiac anomalies. Coarctation of the aorta is a compressed aortic segment made up of localized medial thickening along with a folding inward of the medial and superimposed neointimal tissue. The classic presentation of coarctation of the aorta is in the thoracic aorta below the origin of the left subclavian artery at the aspect of the ductal structure. Poststenotic dilation distal to the segment of coarctation is typically noted. Hypoplasia of the aortic isthmus and the transverse aortic arch is also often present. Collateral circulation may form between the upper body vessels and the vessels distal to the level of coarctation.

Endocardial Cushion Defects

Endocardial cushion defects are also called atrioventricular (AV) canal or septal defects. Endocardial cushion defects may include pathology of the atrial septum, the ventricular septum, and the AV valves. Endocardial cushion defects may be either complete or partial. The complete AV septal defect exhibits both atrial and ventricular septal defects with a common AV valve; a partial defect exhibits an atrial septal defect with distinct mitral and tricuspid valve openings. Endocardial cushion defects cause left-to-right shunting of blood though the heart. A complete endocardial cushion defect may result in volume overload and congestive heart failure.

Supravalvular and Subvalvular Stenosis

Congenital aortic stenosis may be supravalvular, valvular, or subvalvular. Supravalvular aortic stenosis is very rare and is associated with Williams syndrome, which is characterized by hypercalcemia; elfin facies; pulmonary stenosis; aortic hypoplasia; and stenotic renal, celiac, and superior mesenteric arteries. Subvalvular aortic stenosis is associated with hypoplastic left heart syndrome, idiopathic hypertrophic subaortic stenosis, hypertrophic cardiomyopathy, and subaortic fibrous membrane. Subvalvular aortic stenosis is noted in 30% of cases of intrauterine growth restriction. Very few adults present with findings associated with either supravalvular aortic stenosis or subvalvular aortic stenosis; findings are typically the result of a residual postsurgical procedure.

Ventricular Septal Defect

Ventricular septal defect is an opening between the left and right ventricles and is the most typical congenital heart defect in newborns. The presence of a ventricular septal defect results in oxygen-rich blood from the left ventricle being forced into the right ventricle. The subsequent volume overload causes the heart to pump harder and ultimately results in left atrial and left ventricular enlargement. Congestive heart failure may occur as well as pulmonary vascular obstructive disease. Complications of ventricular septal defect may include infective endocarditis, paradoxical emboli, aortic regurgitation, ventricular septum aneurysm, and sudden death.

Marfan's Syndrome

Marfan's syndrome is an inherited connective-tissue disorder that shows up as an autosomal dominant trait. The classic manifestations of Marfan's syndrome are tall stature, ectopia lentis, mitral valve prolapse, dilation of the root of the aorta, and aortic dissection. Dilation of the aorta and aortic dissection are the primary causes of morbidity and mortality. Mitral valve prolapse with a subsequent progression to mitral valve regurgitation is a typical reason for infant morbidity. Without proper treatment, Marfan's syndrome typically results in death at around ages 30 to 40. Most patients with Marfan's syndrome require prophylaxis for endocarditis and beta-blockers.

Indicators of Repaired Congenital Heart Disease

After the repair of congenital heart disease, the following residual effects may be noted: electrophysiological, valvular, vascular, and noncardiovascular. Valvular structural or functional abnormalities after congenital cardiac defect repair may include repaired congenital valve defects that do not function properly, defective valves that were not repaired secondary to normal function, and normal cardiac valves that cannot function properly as a result of the physiologic stress of the defect that necessitated surgery. The ventricles may exhibit residual changes secondary to prior congenital cardiac defect repairs such as ventricular hypertrophy or alterations in left ventricular systolic function.

Clinical Parameters to Note When Evaluating Valve Repair Dysfunction

It is important to note numerous parameters when evaluating valve repair dysfunction with echocardiography. Clinical data should include the date of the valve repair or replacement and the type of valve replacement; the height, weight, and body surface area of the patient; blood pressure and heart rate; and symptoms and clinical findings that are currently present. When imaging the valve repair or replacement, it is critical to note the motion of the leaflets or occluder as well as the presence of calcifications on the valve leaflets or the presence of abnormal densities on the valve itself.

Another crucial parameter to evaluate when imaging for valve repair dysfunction is the integrity of the valve sewing ring and the motion of the repaired valve. Doppler echocardiographic exam should include the contour of the jet velocity signal; the peak velocity and the gradient; the mean pressure gradient; the velocity-time integral of the jet; Doppler velocity index; pressure half-time in the mitral valve and the tricuspid valve; effective orifice area; and the presence, degree, and location of regurgitation. It is also vital to note the size of the left and right ventricles as well as their function, the size of the left and right atria and their function, the presence of any other forms of valve disease, and to estimate the pulmonary artery pressure.

Complications of Systemic Hypertension and Important Echocardiogram Findings

There are numerous complications of systemic hypertension. Some of these complications include coronary artery disease, cerebrovascular accident, renal insufficiency and renal failure, aneurysm, retinopathy, and aortic dissection. There are important M-mode echocardiographic findings in assessing complications of systemic hypertension. M-mode echo findings may include concentric left ventricular hypertrophy, left atrial enlargement, dilation of the root of the aorta, or thickening of the aortic valve that presents as sclerosis as opposed to stenosis. One of the most typical findings on echocardiogram of the complications of systemic hypertension is concentric left ventricular hypertrophy with preservation or enhancement of global systolic function.

Other Echocardiogram Findings of Complications of Systemic Hypertension

Other echocardiogram findings of systemic hypertensive complications that may be demonstrated can be an enlarged left atrium as a result of elevated left ventricular end-diastolic pressure and mitral regurgitation. Decreased left ventricular compliance is demonstrated on echocardiogram by decreased mitral valve E-F slope. Systemic hypertension may result in elevated vascular resistance and increased left ventricular afterload, which ultimately causes left ventricular hypertrophy. Left ventricular hypertrophy subsequently leads to diastolic dysfunction and finally to systolic dysfunction. Left ventricular hypertrophy is a significant risk factor for the future development of adverse cardiac events.

Atrioventricular Septal Defects (AVSDs) in the Adult

Atrioventricular septal defects (AVSDs) used to be called endocardial cushion defects; they demonstrate abnormalities of the septum that is shared between the left ventricle and the right atrium. A complete AVSD is one in which the central aspect of the heart has no atrial or ventricular dividing septal tissue. In this complete AVSD, there will be the presence of a single atrioventricular (AV) valve that enters into both the right and the left ventricle. Every AVSD has two classic features: an absent AV septum and malformed or abnormal atrioventricular heart valves.

Apical Thrombus

The most typical location for a left ventricular thrombus is the apex. Such thrombi are rather difficult to see if the apex is foreshortened; therefore, the use of contrast during echo enables the entire apex to be seen and aids in proper transducer positioning. Echocardiography with contrast will demonstrate a filling defect with the presence of an apical thrombus. Contrast use with echocardiography in the presence of an apical thrombus will typically not demonstrate enhancement, as thrombi are usually avascular in nature. This method is also useful for monitoring the resolution of the thrombus with anticoagulation therapy.

Cardiac Masses and Tumors

Using echocardiography with contrast agents makes it much easier to identify and classify intracardiac masses. An intracardiac mass typically presents as a space-occupying lesion in the cavity of the left ventricle and is frequently not able to be clearly delineated when obtaining baseline views. The administration of an intravenous contrast agent enables one to assess the perfusion status of the mass as well. Typically, malignant masses have abnormal perfusion status as a result of the blood supply needed for rapidly growing tumors. This aspect is usually demonstrated as enhancement of the tumor when compared to surrounding myocardial tissue.

Secondary Cardiac Tumors

Advances in chemotherapy and in radiation therapy has given longer life expectancy to patients with cancer; therefore, the incidence of cardiac metastases has increased to approximately 10%. Many cardiac metastases can be demonstrated with the use of transthoracic and with transesophageal echocardiography. A patient with cancer who develops congestive heart failure, an enlarged heart, or tachyarrhythmia should be considered to have cardiac metastases. Malignant melanoma, malignant germ cell tumors, and malignant thymoma are rare tumors that have a high rate of metastases to the heart. The most common tumors that metastasize to the heart are from the stomach, liver, ovary, colon, and rectum.

Abnormal Cardiac Function as Detected on Echocardiography

The echocardiogram is useful in detecting abnormal cardiac function. The Doppler echocardiogram demonstrates abnormalities in blood flow direction and velocity as an aspect of abnormal cardiac function. Abnormal cardiac function can be exhibited by the size of the chambers of the heart in that the volume or dimension of the chamber may be increased or the chamber walls may be thickened, as is noted with long-standing hypertension. Dilation of the right or left ventricles is an indication of congestive heart failure. Abnormal cardiac function may also be exhibited by a decreased ejection fraction as well.

Abnormal Mitral Valve

The mitral valve is the most complex valve and is frequently associated with abnormal structure and function. Abnormal structure and function of the mitral valve may be stenosis, which causes obstruction to the outflow of blood;

regurgitation, which results in leakage of blood; and prolapse, which allows the valve to bulge backwards. Mitral stenosis results in narrowing of the valve and acts like a dam with subsequent left atrial enlargement. Enlargement of the left atrium may result in electrical disturbances and arrhythmias. Regurgitation may be secondary to enlargement of the left ventricle from long-standing hypertension.

Abnormal Aortic Valve

If the aortic valve is abnormal in structure or in function, congestive heart failure will ultimately develop. Abnormal aortic valve structure and function may also cause infection and sudden death if not properly treated. Aortic stenosis results in the narrowing of the opening of the aortic valve during systole. Aortic stenosis may be secondary to a congenital structural defect of only two cusps as opposed to the normal three cusps of the aortic valve. Aortic stenosis may also be a result of calcium deposition and scarring of the valve cusps and is known as senile degenerative aortic stenosis.

Aortic valve structural abnormalities may result in aortic regurgitation. Aortic regurgitation allows the leakage of blood in a retrograde fashion into the left ventricle during diastole. An enlarged aorta may cause stretching of the cusps of the aortic valve and ultimately result in regurgitation. When aortic regurgitation is present, the left ventricle will compensate for the increased blood volume by dilation and hypertrophy of the walls. Such compensatory measures of the left ventricle allow the heart to pump the blood volume necessary for the body as well as the volume overload that is produced form the retrograde blood flow that is the result of aortic regurgitation.

Abnormal Tricuspid Valve

Tricuspid valve regurgitation may be secondary abnormal dilation of the valve annulus and enlargement of the right ventricle. Such structural abnormalities of the tricuspid valve are frequently the result of left heart failure, right ventricular volume and pressure overload, or dilation of the chambers of the heart. Structural abnormalities of the tricuspid valve may also be caused by congenital defects, rheumatic fever, endocarditis, tricuspid leaflet tear or prolapse, chordal rupture, rupture of a papillary muscle, or myxomatous degeneration of the tricuspid valve. An unusual cause of abnormal tricuspid valve function is pacemaker or defibrillator leads that interrupt the function of the leaflets of the valve.

Abnormal Pulmonary Valve

Most pulmonary valve structural abnormalities are secondary to congenital issues. On occasion, structural and functional abnormalities may be a result of acquired conditions such as carcinoid syndrome or rheumatic fever. Congenital structural abnormalities typically result in stenosis, atresia, or the absence of the leaflets of the pulmonary valve. The typical structural abnormality of the pulmonary valve is that of a dome-shaped valve wherein the leaflets are fused in a cone-like manner and resemble a wind sock. The opening of the pulmonary valve may be anywhere from the size of a pinhole to several millimeters.

Structural abnormalities of the pulmonary valve may include pulmonary valve dysplasia or hypoplasia of the ring of the pulmonary valve ring. Pulmonary valve dysplasia demonstrates thickened, nodular, and redundant leaflets of the valve, which subsequently cause obstruction of blood flow. Hypoplasia of the pulmonary valve ring also results in obstruction of blood flow. Pulmonary valve abnormalities ultimately cause right ventricular hypertrophy that is prominent in the infundibular region. Mild dilation of the cavity of the right ventricle is often noted but may be quite pronounced in cases of severe pulmonary valve stenosis.

Abnormalities of the Pleura

Abnormalities of the pleura are often subtle in appearance. Pneumothorax is an abnormality wherein air becomes trapped in the pleural space. A pneumothorax may occur spontaneously as a consequence of underlying pulmonary disease or as a result of trauma. Pleural thickening may be noted as a result of asbestos exposure with mesothelioma, empyema, pleural effusions, or metastases to the pleura. Pleural plaques present as thickening of the pleura and are typically seen in asbestos exposure. Hemothorax is an abnormality of the pleura wherein blood accumulates in the pleural space and is typically noted after chest trauma.

Abnormalities of the Inferior and Superior Vena Cava

Abnormalities of the inferior and superior vena cava may be congenital or acquired. Examples of congenital abnormalities include persistent left superior vena cava, duplication of the inferior vena cava, and transposition of the inferior vena cava. A persistent left superior vena cava may empty into the left atrium and result in a significant shunt. An acquired abnormality of the superior vena cava is that of superior vena cava syndrome. Superior vena cava syndrome is the result of direct obstruction from malignancy such as right upper lobe tumors, thymoma, or mediastinal lymphadenopathy. Inferior vena cava syndrome is direct obstruction as a result of malignancy or thrombosis.

Clinical Care and Safety

Obtaining Clinical History

It is important to obtain pertinent clinical history from the patient as well as from the medical record. The chief complaint is typically obtained first, and it is the reason that the patient is undergoing the echocardiogram. It is also crucial to ask the patient about the history of the present illness and to review factors such as pain, location, and past medical history. Past medical history obtained from the medical record should include history of congenital heart disease, previous history of myocardial infarction or hypertension, as well as any previous surgical repairs or procedures related to the chief complaint.

Further history that should be obtained from the patient and the medical records includes current medications, medication allergies—especially those related to contrast agents and/or dyes; family history—especially related to congenital heart disease, hypertension, or myocardial infarction; and social history—especially regarding tobacco use and ethanol/drug use. It is also crucial to note pertinent objective findings such as blood pressure, pulse, height, and weight. Other diagnostic data should also be reviewed. Pertinent diagnostic data may include an electrocardiogram (EKG), laboratory studies, x-ray reports—especially chest x-rays, oxygen saturation, Holter monitor/electrophysiology results, operative and/or procedure reports, and any previous echocardiogram study results.

Recording of Diagnostic Observations/Impressions

The diagnostic observations/impressions obtained from the echocardiography study that are to be reported in the patient's medical record should include the cardiac dimensions, assessment of left ventricular ejection fraction, right ventricular systolic pressure, evaluation and assessment of the structure and the function of the anatomic components of the echo exam, a specific evaluation/impression of the presenting problem, and a description of any detected pathological findings. Conclusions should address an overall interpretation and summary of the findings of the study, a diagnostic assessment of the presenting problem, and comparisons to previous echo studies, if available.

It is important to use the lab's internal worksheet in order to organize one's diagnostic observations/impression in order to be thorough in creating the final echocardiographic report. Measurements need to be recorded in the appropriate format and referenced to normal and abnormal values that are typically present on the internal worksheet. It is important to also record visual observations regarding the overall function of the cardiac structures, especially the function of the ventricles and of the valves. A careful description of the impression of the amount of stenosis or regurgitation of the valves is crucial.

Proper Care and Handling of Transducers and Probes

It is important to avoid dropping a transducer, to avoid impact to a transducer, and to prevent abrasion or scratching of a transducer. One should not use a transducer if the housing shaft, acoustic lens, or cable is cracked because this can result in cross-contamination. Cables should be inspected for kinking or excessive twisting. The transducer should be examined for any foreign objects or for the presence of moisture. Dramatic temperature changes may also cause damage to the transducer. The gel to be applied to the acoustic lens of the transducer should be inspected for the presence of any abrasive materials as well.

General Cleaning of a Transducer

General cleaning instructions for transducers are as follows: All soil or other visible contaminants should be wiped from the transducer with a soft cloth before disinfecting. It is critical to wipe off the acoustic gel from the lens before decontamination. Any cleaning product that is used on a transducer should have a neutral pH. The following list of cleaning agents may cause damage: methanol, ethanol, benzyl or methyl alcohol, bleach, methyl or ethyl paraben, polyethylene glycol, mineral oil, lubricant oil, acetone, ammonia, anhydrous ammonia, iodine or iodine compounds, and acids with a pH > 5.

Risk Assessment and Inspection of the Transducer

It is important to always inspect the transducer prior to each use for mechanical or electrical hazards. A transducer that is damaged can cause injury to a patient or contribute to a greater risk of infection. A visual inspection needs to be performed to assess for sharp, pointed, or rough damage to the surface of the transducer that could result in injury to a patient or damage to a protective transducer cover such as a glove or a sheath. The transducer should also be inspected for any type of damage that may increase the risk of electrical shock, especially if conductive solutions are used.

Overview of Anaphylactoid Reactions to Contrast Agents

Anaphylactoid reactions to contrast agents exhibit manifestations identical to anaphylactic reactions but are not mediated by an allergen-IgE complex. Anaphylactoid reactions may happen even if first-time contrast is given; the extent and severity of the reaction is not related to dose; thus, a test dose is of no utility. Risk factors include allergic asthma, drug allergies, food allergies, and previous contrast reactions. Symptoms of life-threatening reaction include laryngeal edema, arrhythmias, seizures, severe hypotension, unresponsiveness, and cardiac arrest. The presence of these symptoms necessitates immediate treatment.

Treatment of Anaphylactoid Reactions to Contrast Agents

It is imperative to have an emergency crash cart readily available. The crash cart should have appropriate emergency medications, bag valve mask, oxygen, endotracheal tubes, intravenous (IV) solutions such as lactated Ringer's or normal saline, IV tubing, needles, syringes, masks, airways, laryngoscopes, blood pressure cuff, and stethoscopes. The infusion of contrast agent must be stopped immediately.

IV fluid should be started and run wide open. Vital signs and airway assessment are to be obtained. Administer oxygen by mask at 6 to 10 liters per minute, and intubate with a laryngoscope and endotracheal tube if the airway may be compromised.

Medications Used to Treat Anaphylactoid Reactions to Contrast Agents

Numerous medications may be used to treat reactions to contrast agents. Common medications include the following: albuterol inhaler to reduce bronchospasm and facilitate bronchodilator; atropine to treat bradycardia from a vasovagal reaction (characterized by slow heart rate and hypotension); diphenhydramine (H_1 receptor blocker) to block histamine from binding to target cells and is most efficacious for mild urticaria; clonidine for hypertensive crisis; epinephrine, an alpha-agonist, to treat profound urticaria, facial edema, and laryngeal edema; the beta-2 agonist properties of epinephrine to treat bronchospasm; diazepam to treat seizures; and nitroglycerin for acute angina.

Maintenance of Training in Basic Life Support Techniques

It is essential to maintain current certification in basic life support techniques because the adult cardiac patient is at risk for myocardial infarction, congestive heart failure, cardiac arrhythmia, or sudden death. In addition, the use of contrast agents or various medications may cause an allergic or anaphylactic reaction. A severe allergic reaction or anaphylactic reaction may result in severe hypotension, bradycardia, and even cardiac arrest. Basic life support is a first-line measure to maintain circulation and respiration while preparing or opening the crash cart to obtain intravenous setups, medications, airways, and other equipment for resuscitation.

Measurement Techniques, Maneuvers, and Sonographic Views

Analyzing Right Ventricular Size and Systolic Function

Echocardiography is a useful tool to evaluate right ventricular size and function in a qualitative manner. The right ventricle should be similar in size to the left ventricle; the right ventricle should be about two-thirds the size of the left ventricle upon the parasternal long axis and apical four-chamber views. If the right ventricle looks larger than the left ventricle, right ventricular dilation may be suspected. In the short-axis views, the right ventricle is smaller than the left ventricle and the left ventricle appears circular during the course of the cardiac cycle.

Measurement Techniques for Right Ventricle Systolic Function

Right ventricle systolic function may be assessed by using multiple means, including right ventricular index of myocardial performance (RIMP), tricuspid annular plane systolic excursion (TAPSE), two-dimensional right ventricular fractional area change (2D RV FAC), 2D RV ejection fraction, three-dimensional right ventricular ejection fraction (3D RV EF), tissue Doppler-derived tricuspid lateral annular systolic velocity (S′), and longitudinal strain and strain rate. RIMP demonstrates a global index for right ventricular function. TAPSE is used to demonstrate RV longitudinal function. 2D RV FAC yields an estimate of the function of the right ventricle in systole.

Quantification of the Left Atrium from 2D Images

The size of the left atrium is determined by measuring the end-ventricular systole when the left atrium chamber is at its greatest size. The left atrial base needs to be at its maximal size, which is an indication that the plane of imaging goes through the maximal short-axis area. The volume of the left atrium has often been calculated by using a cube formula; studies have demonstrated that this method is not as reliable as other methods of calculation. Research has shown that the most accurate calculation of left atrial volume is obtained with an ellipsoid model or with Simpson's rule.

Measurement of Left Ventricle Chamber Size and Wall Thickness from 2D Images

The parasternal long-axis acoustical window should be used in order to get the most accurate linear measurements of interventricular septal and posterior wall thicknesses as well as the most accurate measurement of the interior dimension of the left ventricle. It is important to assess the interior dimensions of the left ventricle and the thicknesses of the septal and posterior walls at the period of end-diastole and end-systole during the course of several cardiac cycles. It is now feasible to assess the actual thickness of the ventricular septum and other chambers by using the true blood–tissue interface.

Measurement of the Aorta from 2D Images

The parasternal long-axis acoustic window is used to assess the root of the aorta and the proximal ascending aorta. Locations for measurements should be obtained from the annulus of the aortic valve, the greatest diameter in the sinuses of Valsalva, and at the sinotubular junction (the area between the sinuses of Valsalva and the tubular aspect of the ascending aorta). Echocardiographic views need to be such that the greatest diameter of the aortic root is ascertained. There is a strong correlation between the diameter of the aortic root at the sinuses of Valsalva and body surface and age.

Measurement of the Inferior Vena Cava from 2D Images

The inferior vena cava diameter is typically accurately measured with a patient in a left decubitus position approximately 1 to 2 cm from the junction with the right atrium by means of the long-axis view. The values that are obtained need to be from measurements that are perpendicular to the long axis of the inferior vena cava. The inferior vena cava diameter becomes smaller during inspiration as a consequence of the negative intrathoracic pressure, causing greater right ventricular filling from the systemic veins. Right atrial pressure, therefore, correlates with the inferior vena cava diameter and the amount of decrease in diameter in inspiration (collapsibility index).

M-Mode Images

Cardiac imaging typically involves three basic modes: 2D, M-mode, and Doppler. M-mode echocardiography yields a one-dimensional view and is typically used for fine measurements. The M-mode is also known as the motion mode and is frequently used to evaluate the motion of the cardiac valves, the sizes of the cardiac chambers, the size of the root of the aorta, the thicknesses of the walls, and the function of the ventricles. A slender ultrasound beam that is sent in a single plane through the heart and produces images of the tissue in that plane with a very high temporal and spatial resolution is known as the M-mode.

Assessment of the Ejection Fraction by 2D Measurements

The ejection fraction is a key component to consider when assessing cardiac function. The ejection fraction is a key determinant of the quantity of blood pumped from the ventricles. The ejection fraction is commonly determined by Simpson's rule. Simpson's rule serves to approximate the left ventricle by means of a stack of circular (or elliptical) discs whose centers are all in the major axis. The area-length method is used for symmetrical left ventricles, and it is the area of the left ventricle squared and divided by the length and multiplied by 0.85.

Diastolic Function Assessment

Using Left Ventricular Inflow

The most typical method to assess left ventricular diastolic function is that of pulsed-wave Doppler of left ventricular inflow across the mitral valve in diastole. The cursor of the Doppler is situated at the tips of the mitral leaflets in the apical four-chamber view. A normal left ventricle will demonstrate an early wave (E wave), which reflects the majority of filling that happens in early diastole. The A wave represents atrial systole and has a slower velocity than the E wave. An E:A wave ratio of greater than 1 is considered normal.

Using Pulmonary Venous Flow

Pulmonary venous flow can be ascertained by pulsed-wave Doppler in the apical four-chamber view and is a useful means to determine diastolic function. The transducer should be situated so that the aortic valve is demonstrated. The measurements of pulmonary venous waveforms include peak systolic velocity (S), peak antegrade diastolic velocity (D), the S/D ratio, systolic filling fraction, and the peak Ar velocity in late diastole. There are two systolic velocities: S1 reflects the relaxation of the atria, and S2 is used to calculate the ratio of the peak systolic to the peak diastolic velocity.

Using Tissue Doppler or Color Doppler

The typical methods used in tissue Doppler to evaluate diastolic function depend upon patterns of mitral inflow. The velocity across the mitral valve is directly correlated to preload (left atrial pressure) and independently and inversely correlated to the relaxation of the ventricle. The velocity across the mitral valve demonstrates the pressure gradient that exists between the left atrium and the left ventricle. The assessment of diastolic function using tissue Doppler does not depend as much on load as does regular Doppler. "Ea" represents the early myocardial relaxation velocity and may be exhibited anywhere on the mitral annulus.

Using Isovolumetric Relaxation Time

Dr. Carl J. Wiggers defines the onset of isovolumetric relaxation time as "aortic valve closure which can be readily determined from cusp apposition of the M-mode echocardiogram, the closure artifact on an aortic Doppler, or A2, the aortic component of the second sound on a phonocardiogram, which are all effectively synchronous." Isovolumetric relaxation time can be readily obtained by Doppler echocardiography. A prolonged isovolumetric relaxation time represents abnormal myocardial relaxation as the pressure in the left ventricle declines slowly during the isovolumetric relaxation phase, which causes a delay in the time before the left ventricular pressure declines below the left atrial pressure.

High Pulse Repetition Frequency (PRF)

Pulsed-wave Doppler that has been modified for high pulse repetition frequency (PRF) is a measurement technique that is used to record high flow velocities. High pulse repetition frequency uses range ambiguity to elevate the maximum velocity that can be ascertained by pulsed-wave Doppler. Numerous sample volumes are situated proximal to the area and at the location of the area to be studied. The depth of the proximal sample will serve to ascertain the high pulse repetition frequency. The high pulse repetition frequency enables determination of higher velocities at the area to be studied that are not compromised by signal aliasing.

Color and Spectral Doppler

Spectral analysis display or spectral Doppler occurs when a transducer obtains backscattered sound waves, which have analysis of their frequencies and subsequent comparison to the transmitted signal frequencies. The display demonstrates time on a midline horizontal axis and frequencies on a vertical axis. The frequency signal is demonstrated as a pixel on the vertical axis; the grayscale represents amplitude, and the location on the vertical axis represents the velocity of blood flow. Color Doppler is a form of pulsed-wave Doppler that enables evaluation of numerous samples along numerous sampling lines in color instead of in grayscale.

Tissue Doppler Imaging

Doppler tissue imaging is a type of pulsed-wave Doppler that allows measurement of cardiac motion and velocity. Pulsed-wave Doppler uses a filter to prevent lower velocities created by cardiac tissue; tissue Doppler does not use this filter and therefore is able to ascertain high-amplitude, low-velocity signals created by tissue motion. Global assessment is accomplished by putting a 1-cm-length sample volume at the mitral annulus, while regional assessment is accomplished by placing the 1-cm-long sample within the cardiac tissues. Tissue Doppler may also be used to evaluate longitudinal and radial ventricular contraction.

PISA Measurements to Evaluate Valvular Lesions

The proximal isovelocity surface area (PISA) method is also known as flow convergence. It is based on the hemodynamic principle that states as blood comes into a regurgitant orifice, its velocity increases, forming concentric, roughly hemispheric shells of increasing velocity and decreasing surface area. Color flow mapping can be used to demonstrate an image of one of the hemispheres, which relates to the Nyquist limit. If a Nyquist limit is obtained, in which the flow convergence appears like a hemisphere, the flow rate is the product of the surface area of the hemisphere and the aliasing velocity.

Calculation of Regurgitant Fractions

The stroke volume (SV) at the valve annulus is the product of the cross-sectional area and the velocity time interval (VTI) at the annulus: SV = CSA X VTI = pi X diameter squared/4 X VTI = 0.785 X diameter squared X VTI. CSA, cross-sectional area of the left ventricular outflow tract. The stroke volume may be derived from two or more areas and should be equal if there is no regurgitation. Regurgitation in one valve will exhibit a larger amount of flow than the competent valves. The regurgitant volume is the difference between the two valves. According to the American Society of Echocardiography, the regurgitant fraction is "regurgitant volume divided by the forward stroke volume through the regurgitant valve." $RV = SV_{\text{regurgitant valve}} - SV_{\text{competent valve}}$. $RF = (SV_{\text{regurgitant valve}} - SV_{\text{competent valve}})/SV_{\text{regurgitant valve}}$.

Calculation of Shunt Ratios

The echocardiogram may be used to estimate the size of a left-to-right or right-to-left shunt. Shunt ratios are typically calculated as the ratio of pulmonic blood flow

(Qp) to the systemic blood flow (Qs). A ratio > 1 typically demonstrates a left-to-right shunt, whereas a ratio < 1 demonstrates a right-to-left shunt. To calculate the shunt ratio, the stroke volume at the left ventricular outflow tract is used to estimate the left side while the right side is measured at the right ventricular outflow tract. It is important to recall that the ratio is very sensitive to measurement errors of the diameters of the left ventricular outflow tract (LVOT) and right ventricular outflow tract (RVOT).

Calculation of Mitral Valve Area

Using 2D Planimetry

2D planimetry is a reference measurement for the area of the mitral valve: it is considered to be a direct measurement of the area of the mitral valve and does not require using hypotheses about flow conditions, the compliance of the chambers of the heart, or associated lesions of the valves. To perform 2D planimetry, the opening of the mitral valve is traced in the parasternal short-axis view. The plane of the measurement needs to be perpendicular to the opening of the mitral valve. Two-dimensional planimetry should be undertaken during mid-diastole of the cardiac cycle.

Using the Pressure Half-Time Method

T ½ is defined as the interval of time in milliseconds between the maximal mitral gradient in early diastole and the time where the gradient is half the maximum initial value. The decline of the velocity of diastolic transmitral blood flow is inversely proportional to valve area (centimeters squared). The mitral valve area (MVA) = 220/T ½. T ½ is determined by a tracing of the deceleration slope of the E wave on Doppler spectral display of the transmitral flow. The area of the valve is typically then automatically figured by the software of the echocardiogram machine.

Using Continuity Equation

The theory of conservation of mass is the basis for the continuity equation. The continuity equation demonstrates that the filling volume in diastole of the mitral flow is equal to the aortic stroke volume. MVA = (pi) (diameter squared/4) ($VTI_{aortic}/VTI_{mitral}$), where VTI is the velocity time interval. The diameter in this equation is the diameter of the left ventricular outflow tract in centimeters; VTI is also in centimeters. It can be difficult to obtain accuracy and reproducibility of the continuity equation secondary to the number of measurements necessary, which serves to increase the impact of measurement errors. Atrial fibrillation or significant mitral/aortic regurgitation prevents the use of this equation.

Using the Proximal Isovelocity Surface Area Method

The formula for the calculation of mitral valve area (MVA) using the proximal isovelocity surface area (PISA) method is MVA = (pi) (radius squared) ($V_{aliasing}$)/peak V_{mitral} X a/180 degrees. The radius of the convergence hemisphere is measured in centimeters, $V_{aliasing}$ is the aliasing velocity measured in centimeters per second, the peak V_{mitral} is the color-wave Doppler velocity of mitral inflow measured in centimeters per second, and a is the opening angle of the mitral leaflets relative to the direction of blood flow. The PISA method is useful in the arena of significant mitral regurgitation, but it is difficult to perform accurately.

Calculation of Aortic Valve Areas

Using the Continuity Equation When Stenosis Is Present

When stenosis of the valve is present, the area of the aortic valve (AVA) can be calculated with the continuity equation as the stroke volume that is ejected via the left ventricular outflow tract all goes through the stenotic opening of the aortic valve; therefore, the stroke volume is equal at both sites. The equation is $AVA = (CSA_{LVOT} \times VTI_{LVOT}) / VTI_{aortic\ valve}$. CSA, cross-sectional area of the left ventricular outflow tract; LVOT, left ventricular outflow tract; VTI, velocity time interval. The continuity equation uses the following measurements: jet velocity of aortic stenosis determined by color-wave Doppler, LVOT diameter to calculate CSA, and LVOT velocity (recorded with pulsed Doppler).

Using 2D Planimetry

2D planimetry uses direct measurement by visualization of the opening of the aortic valve in the course of either 2D or 3D transthoracic echo or transesophageal echo. Two-dimensional planimetry may be helpful if Doppler estimation of velocities of flow is not accurate or reliable. Planimetry can be unreliable, however, when calcification of the valve is present. Calcification of the valve may result in the presence of shadows or reverberations that hamper the correct identification of the opening of the aortic valve. When using 2D planimetry, one must ensure that the minimal orifice area is correctly identified.

Quantification of the Severity of Mitral Valve Regurgitant

In order to quantify the severity of mitral valve regurgitation, it is important to assess the structure of the mitral valve and to evaluate the hemodynamic effects of mitral regurgitation on the left atrium and the left ventricle. It is critical to carefully outline the entire mitral valve structure; the most typical structural abnormality noted is that of myxomatous degeneration of the valve. It is also crucial to assess the hemodynamic effects on the left atrium and the left ventricle. Enlargement of the left atrium is often noted as well as dilation of the left ventricle as a result of volume overload.

Quantification of the Severity of Aortic Valve Regurgitation

A combination of echocardiography, spectral Doppler, and color Doppler is necessary to best quantify the severity of aortic valve regurgitation. The usual method of echocardiography does not directly visualize aortic regurgitation; aortic regurgitation is typically inferred from the demonstration of high-frequency fluttering of the anterior mitral valve leaflet or of the interventricular septum using the M-mode. It is important to assess the impact of aortic regurgitation on the left ventricle when quantifying aortic regurgitation. Volume overload as a result of aortic regurgitation will result in dilation of the left ventricle with a decrease in ejection fraction.

Changing the Sample Volume Size

One of the advantages of using pulsed-wave Doppler is the provision of Doppler shift data in a selective manner from a small segment of the ultrasound beam, which is also known as the sample volume. The operator is in control of the location of the sample volume. Ultrasound speed in tissues is constant; thus, there is a direct relationship between the entire travel time of the ultrasound pulse and the sample volume location relative to the transducer. The operator may choose specific locations for the sample volume size based on a timing mechanism.

Quantifying the Left Atrial Volume

Emerging evidence demonstrates that enlargement of the left atrium is a strong predictor in outcomes of cardiac disease. Recent studies have shown that the volume of the left atrium is much more accurate in measuring the size of the left atrium than using the M-mode to assess the dimensions of the left atrium. The American Society of Echocardiography suggests using biplane 2D echocardiography with the disc method (Simpson's rule) or the area-length method to assess the left atrium size. Maximum and minimum left atrial volume reference values are 22 ± 6 ml/m^2 and 9 ± 4 ml/m^2.

Quantifying the Left Ventricular Systolic Function

The ejection fraction of the left ventricle is typically the best method to quantify left ventricular systolic function. The ejection fraction is determined by the difference between end-diastolic volume and end-systolic left ventricular volume divided by the end-diastolic left ventricular volume. The left ventricular volumes are usually obtained via the 2D biplane method of discs also known as Simpson's rule. The left ventricular volumes are obtained from apical four-chamber and/or apical two-chamber views. An accurate tracing of the endocardial border of the left ventricle is essential; measurements of the diastolic and systolic volumes have to be taken during the same cardiac cycle.

Structures on Echocardiogram That May Be Misinterpreted as Cardiac Masses or Tumors

It is important to be able to distinguish between normal cardiac structures that may resemble a mass and pathologic cardiac masses or tumors on echocardiogram. The following normal structures and variants may be mistaken for a cardiac mass or tumor. (1) Right atrium: Chiari network, Eustachian valve, crista terminalis, catheters or pacemaker leads, pectinate muscles, fatty hypertrophy of the interatrial septum, and fatty deposits around the tricuspid annulus. (2) Left atrium: heart transplant suture lines, fossa ovalis, calcified mitral valve annulus, coronary sinus, and transverse sinus. (3) Right ventricle: moderator band, muscle bundles, and catheters/pacemaker leads. (4) Left ventricle: false chords, papillary muscles, and left ventricular trabeculations.

Standard Adult Echocardiogram Report as Suggested by the ASE

According to the Task Force of the American Society of Echocardiography (ASE) on Recommendations for a Standardized Report for Adult Transthoracic

Echocardiography, the following sections should be present: demographic and other identifying information, echocardiographic evaluation, and summary. Demographic and other identifying information may include the age, gender, height, weight, and blood pressure of the patient as well as the location of the media for the echo study, date of the study, location of the patient and the location where the study was performed, the name of the ordering physician, and the technician performing the study.

Cardiac and Vascular Structures That Are Typically Evaluated and That Should Be Included

As outlined in the American Society of Echocardiography (ASE) task force recommendations, typical cardiac and vascular structures examined in an adult transthoracic echocardiogram include the left ventricle, left atrium, right atrium, right ventricle, aortic valve, mitral valve, tricuspid valve, pulmonic valve, pericardium, aorta, pulmonary artery, inferior vena cava and pulmonary veins. Measurements are an important element of the comprehensive echocardiogram report as well. Quantitative measurements are preferred; however, qualitative and semiquantitative measurements are frequently used and may be thought to be appropriate/adequate. Measurements may include dimension, wall thickness, and function, severity of stenosis or regurgitation, and the presence of and severity of cardiac shunts.

Descriptive Statements and Summary in an Echocardiogram Report

According to American Society of Echocardiography (ASE) task force recommendations, descriptive statements may be broad in nature and may be modified to fit the nature of the study. An example would be a description of the cavity size of the left ventricle using the following terms: normal, increased (mild, moderate, severe), or decreased. Ventricular shape may be described as normal, concentric hypertrophy (mild, moderate, severe), asymmetric hypertrophy (absent, present-anterior, posterior, septal, lateral, apical, basal), eccentric hypertrophy (absent, present), and aneurysm. The summary should include answers to question posed for the study, an emphasis on abnormal results, and a comparison to previous studies, if applicable.

Incorporation of Outside Data in an Echocardiogram Report

A typical echocardiogram (echo) report should include incorporation of outside data that is obtained from the patient's clinical history as well as the patient's medical records. Data to be obtained may include the patient's height, weight, derived body surface area, heart rate, blood pressure, and cardiac rhythm. Such information is helpful when interpreting structural and functional quantitative data on echo. The patient's blood pressure measurements are typically needed in the case of conditions such as aortic regurgitation or mitral regurgitation, which may affect afterload and thus echocardiographic results. Clinical data on the current condition of the patient are also necessary for echo interpretation.

2D Echocardiogram Findings in Pulmonary Hypertension

The 2D echocardiogram may demonstrate an etiology of the underlying cause of pulmonary hypertension such as ischemic cardiac disease. Right ventricular hypertrophy and right ventricular dilation is also noted. The right ventricle forms a cardiac apex, which is indicative of dilation of the right ventricle. The left ventricle appears D-shaped as a result of a leftward shift of the interventricular septum. Another 2D echocardiogram finding of pulmonary hypertension is dilation of the inferior vena cava and hepatic veins and the failure of the inferior vena cava to collapse 50% or more with inspiration.

Systolic Pulmonary Artery Pressure Derivation and the Severity Scale

The following formula is used to determine the systolic pulmonary artery pressure: sPAP (mm Hg) = 1.23 X (Vmax TR squared) – 0.09 mm Hg. Normal sPAP is 18 to 25 mm Hg. Mild severity is sPAP of 30 to 40 mm Hg. Moderate severity is indicated by sPAP of 40 to 70 mm Hg. Severe is sPAP of greater than 70 mm Hg. Eisenmenger's syndrome is the presence of severe pulmonary hypertension and congenital heart disease with an occurrence of a reversal of a left-to-right shunt and typically has sPAP > 120 mm Hg.

Echocardiogram in Evaluation of Arrhythmias and Conduction Disturbances

Echocardiography is primarily used to assess for underlying cardiac disease as a possible cause of arrhythmias or conduction disturbances. Identification of underlying cardiac disease can aid in guiding the treatment and prognosis of the arrhythmia or the conduction disturbance. Typically, echocardiography is useful in evaluating patients with atrial fibrillation, atrial flutter, reentrant tachycardia, ventricular tachycardia, and ventricular fibrillation. An echocardiographic exam also will enable an assessment of cardiac function in the setting of an arrhythmia or conduction disturbance. An echocardiogram is a valuable test in the workup of an arrhythmia or conduction disturbance prior to performing ablation as well.

Echocardiography in the Identification and Evaluation of Atrial Septal Defect in the Adult

Atrial septal defects are classified based upon the location of the defect: ostium secundum, ostium primum, sinus venosus, and coronary sinus defects. Atrial septal defects result in shunting from the left atrium to the right atrium; large shunts will cause enlargement of the right atrium and the right ventricle as a consequence of increased volume. Secundum defects are located in the center of the atrial septum and are enclosed on all sides by atrial septal tissue. Ostium primum defects are located adjacent to the atrioventricular valves. In the subcostal view, a classic hallmark is the absence of the atrial septum next to the AV valves.

It is crucial to recall that a primum defect may go into an atrioventricular valve leaflet. An example would be a cleft mitral valve. The parasternal short axis view will demonstrate two anterior mitral valve leaflets because the primum defect extends into anterior mitral leaflet. The presence of a cleft mitral valve may indicate a cause of mitral regurgitation. Sinus venosus defects will be best shown using a subcostal long-axis view of the inferior and superior vena cavae because these defects are situated superiorly on the interatrial septum adjacent to its junction with the superior vena cava.

Ventricular Septal Defects (VSDs) in the Adult

The ventricular septum is usually divided into the following three components: subarterial, perimembranous, and muscular. If there is a large shunt as a result of a ventricular septal defect (VSD), the right ventricle will enlarge significantly, and the pressures in the left and right side of the heart will become equal. Doppler echo is quite helpful in the identification of large or small VSDs. Muscular VSDs are typically surrounded by areas of muscular septum. Subarterial VSDs are also known as outlet VSDs and are located below arteries.

Echocardiography with Contrast Identification of Aortic Dissection

Transesophageal echocardiography is considered the gold standard for imaging suspected aortic dissection; however, contrast echocardiography is very useful when it is difficult to demonstrate the intimal flap or to delineate an intimal flap from an artifact. The use of contrast with echocardiography will also enable the determination of a true lumen versus a false lumen. On occasion, the use of echocardiogram contrast may be helpful in the determination of the entry or exit point of the dissection as well as determining if the dissection plane has gone into any major branches of the aorta.

Pericardiocentesis

Pericardiocentesis is the aspiration of fluid from the pericardial space that surrounds the heart. Echocardiography is a standard imaging modality in the assessment of pericardial effusions and cardiac tamponade because it enables estimation of the size of the effusion and the hemodynamic consequences. Assessment of hemodynamic effects include abnormal septal motion, inversion of the right atrium or right ventricle, and diminished respiratory variation of the diameter of the inferior vena cava. Emergent pericardiocentesis is performed when life-threatening hemodynamics are present, while nonemergent pericardiocentesis is used to obtain fluid for diagnostic, palliative, or prophylactic measures.

There are no absolute contraindications for emergent pericardiocentesis; relative contraindications include an uncorrected bleeding diathesis or traumatic cardiac tamponade. The technique is as follows: identify the xiphoid process; needle insertion is typically performed at the left sternocostal margin or subxiphoid; local anesthetic is used before a # 11 blade is used to puncture the skin; a 20- or 60-ml syringe is connected to a spinal needle, and 5 cc of normal saline is aspirated into the syringe; the spinal needle is inserted and directed toward the left shoulder; negative pressure is maintained until fluid return or cardiac pulsations are noted; and the needle is removed upon no further aspiration of fluid.

Instrumentation, Optimization, and Contrast

Ultrasound Imaging Artifacts

Even high-quality studies may exhibit ultrasound artifacts. Ultrasound imaging artifacts may be thought to be pathologic. An example would be near-field clutter and reverberations on 2D echo that are confused with apical thrombi. Other examples of ultrasound imaging artifacts may be secondary to obesity, chronic obstructive pulmonary disease, pneumothorax, subcutaneous emphysema, and even bowel gas as a result of the air interface. Some other imaging artifacts include acoustic shadows, edge shadows, and acoustic enhancement. Some structures may appear more echogenic as a result of the posterior enhancement effect; shadowing artifacts and edge artifacts are also problematic.

Appearance of Common Ultrasound Imaging Artifacts

Reverberation is an ultrasound imaging artifact that appears as bright parallel lines that happen at regular intervals. The reverberation pseudomass is usually the result of returned echoes from a gas- or fluid-filled structure in a location that is deep to the transducer. The closer wall of the pseudomass is secondary to primary reflection from the tissue/gas or fluid interface, while the far wall is a result of the reverberated echo. Partial attenuation of the sound wave may be the result of absorption, reflection, or refraction and appear to be an area of low echogenicity.

Mirror-image pseudomasses may be found near highly reflective acoustic interfaces as a result of reverberations that occur between a true mass and a reflective surface. The presence of a mirror-image pseudomass above the diaphragm is always an artifact. Refraction artifacts can be mistaken as shadowing from calcification, or they may limit assessment of tissue in the region of the artifact. Side-lobe artifacts are low-intensity sound beams that are found peripheral to the primary axis of the ultrasound beam. When side-lobe artifacts interact with a highly reflective acoustic surface, significant specular or diffuse echoes may result.

Using a Respirometer to Evaluate Cardiac Constriction

In constrictive pericarditis, there is a demonstrated dissociation between intracardiac and intrathoracic pressures. Normally, there is a decline in intracardiac and intrathoracic pressures with inspiration. In constrictive pericarditis, the decline in intrathoracic pressure is not transmitted to the left side of the heart; therefore, the left ventricle is not filled properly during inspiration secondary to the lower pulmonary pressure. Also, both the right and left ventricles have enhanced interaction as they are using the same space. The left ventricle is not filled adequately in inspiration, and the right ventricle exhibits overfilling. During expiration, the right ventricle is underfilled, while the left ventricle is overfilled.

Findings with a Respirometer with Cardiac Tamponade

Reciprocal changes are demonstrated in the right and the left ventricles during respiration. Such changes represent interdependence of the ventricles. With inspiration, the interventricular septum protrudes into the left ventricle as a result of elevated systemic venous return to the right ventricle. The limited expansion of the free wall of the right ventricle secondary to elevated intrapericardial pressure also contributes to the protrusion of the interventricular septum into the left ventricle. With expiration, the transmitral pressure gradient is elevated; the systemic venous return declines, and diastolic flow reversal occurs in the hepatic veins.

Analysis of dP/dT

The rate of pressure change during contraction is represented by dP/dT and may be demonstrated in a noninvasive manner by the continuous-wave Doppler mitral regurgitation velocity curve. An analysis of dP/dT may be used as an indicator of the function of the left ventricle. The mitral regurgitant dP/dT is not dependent on afterload but is influenced by preload as this serves as a measurement of the left ventricular contractibility during the isovolumetric contraction phase. The apical four-chamber view is used, and identification of the mitral regurgitant jet is accomplished with color flow imaging. Points at one second and at three seconds are marked, with the time interval between the two points noted as Ti. $dP/dT = 32/Ti$.

Provocative Maneuvers in Echocardiography

Provocative maneuvers are useful in echocardiography to aid in improving image quality and also to aid in diagnosing certain pathologic conditions. Expiration may be used to improve the 2D echo image because it facilitates greater parasternal and apical access to the heart. Inspiration may be used to improve the 2D echo image because it causes the diaphragm to descend, which improves access to the heart. In order to limit excessive translation of the heart during the use of M-mode measurements of left ventricular function, quiet respiration withheld end-expiration is useful.

End-expiratory apnea is a useful maneuver to limit excessive translation of the heart when obtaining Doppler flow or tissue velocities. Inspiration or a brief sniff is useful when obtaining an estimate of right atrial pressures because this maneuver creates the inspiratory response of the inferior vena cava to facilitate determination of the collapsibility index. Normal inspiration and expiration are performed in order to ascertain the respiratory variation in the systolic forward flow in the superior vena cava; this technique may be used to evaluate the systolic pulmonary artery pressure in the presence of chronic obstructive pulmonary disease.

The typical Valsalva maneuver may be used to ascertain left ventricular diastolic function for the following reasons: to reveal elevated left ventricular filling pressure in patients with normal or reduced left ventricular systolic function and a pseudonormal filling pattern at baseline (secondary to the decrease in the mitral E/A ratio of 0.5 or more during Valsalva) and in patients with a weakened relaxation pattern at baseline (as a result of the increase in peak A-wave velocity during Valsalva). The Valsalva maneuver may also be used in detection of a patent foramen ovale and in hypertrophic cardiomyopathy.

Estimation of Pulmonary Artery Systolic Pressure

The pulmonary artery systolic pressure is nearly equivalent to the right ventricular pressure if no right ventricular outflow obstruction is present. The pulmonary artery systolic pressure and thus the right ventricular pressure may be calculated as follows: tricuspid regurgitant jet is a reflection of the maximum pressure gradient between the right atrium and the right ventricle during systole, and the simplified Bernoulli equation is used to calculate the peak pressure gradient with the peak tricuspid velocity. The right ventricular and pulmonary artery systolic pressures are then estimated by adding the peak pressure gradient to the right atrial pressure.

Estimation of Right Atrial Pressure

The pressure of the right atrium may be estimated by taking the measurement of the dimensions of the inferior vena cava (IVC) and its collapse upon inspiration using the following steps: the patient is placed in the left lateral decubitus position; a subcostal view is used to visualize the IVC draining into the right atrium; the IVC needs to be visualized in a long-axis view; the IVC should be measured 1 to 2 cm within the junction of the IVC and right atrium; the maximum and minimum diameters are obtained; and the collapsibility index is then calculated.

Correlation of Pressure Gradients and the Severity of Valve Stenosis

The mean pressure gradient may be used to classify the severity of valve stenosis. According to the American Heart Association/American College of Cardiology guidelines, aortic stenosis is mild at less than 20 mm Hg, moderate at 20 to 40 mm Hg, and severe at greater than 40 mm Hg. Mitral stenosis is classified as mild at a mean pressure gradient of less than 5 mm Hg, moderate at a mean pressure gradient between 5 to 10 mm Hg, and severe at a mean pressure gradient greater than 10 mm Hg. Tricuspid stenosis is significant at a mean pressure gradient greater than or equal to 5 mm Hg. Pulmonic stenosis is mild at < 36 mm, moderate at 36 to 64 mm, and severe at > 64 mm Hg.

Use of Color Doppler as an Integral Part of the Doppler Exam

Color Doppler is quite helpful in providing information about the direction of blood flow, velocity, and flow patterns. Flow patterns may be laminar or turbulent. Color Doppler imaging will demonstrate blood flow as color-coded velocities superimposed on the 2D or M-mode in real time. Color Doppler is typically based on the BART scale: blue away, red toward. For example, an apical four-chamber color Doppler view will demonstrate blue flow along the left ventricular outflow tract in early systole that moves away from the transducer and red flow toward the apex or transducer.

Adjustment for PRF

It is important to recall that the number of pulses per second, also known as the pulse repetition frequency (PRF), is related to the maximum time of travel and the depth of imaging. For each scan line, the PRF will be the determinant of the frame rate. The frame rate is the number of images created per second and stored in memory. The greater the depth of the image is, the lower the PRF and therefore the lower the frame rate. More scan lines will lower the frame rate.

Adjustment of Dynamic Range

Dynamic range serves to control the contrast of an image. Dynamic range may be automatically adjusted by an echocardiographic machine or may be manually adjusted by an echocardiography technician. It is important to recall that the dynamic range control is used in order to ascertain a correct range to be displayed as a result of a wide range of echo signals. Typically, the displayed range is an eight-bit black-and-white image obtained from a wide range of log-compressed echo signal. If the value of the dynamic range is changed, the image contrast can be adjusted.

Adjustment of the Focal Zone

The focal zone of the transducer is the area wherein the beam narrows. Typically, the intensity of the ultrasound can be increased 100 times or more when compared to the intensity located outside the focal zone. As a result of the elevated intensity, a greater signal will be created in the transducer from a reflector that is located in the focal zone. The focal zone also corresponds to the area of the best lateral resolution. The focus will need to be adjusted appropriately to the level of interest of the exam. Multiple focal zones are typically present on most machines.

Adjustment of Pre- or Postprocessing Parameters

If adjustment of pre- or postprocessing parameters is needed, it is crucial to remember the three categories of Doppler controls. The first category of controls is the group that will influence the quality of the recording. These controls are gain, gray scale, and wall filter. The second category of controls is the group that alters the appearance of the graphic display. These controls are the scale factor and baseline position. The last category of controls is the group that is primarily used in pulsed-wave Doppler as they correlate sample volume. These controls are cursor, sample depth, and angle.

Using Contrast for Left Ventricular or Doppler Enhancement

The American Society of Echocardiography (ASE) has recommended the use of contrast "for the purposes of improving endocardial visualization in all subjects with > 2 suboptimal contiguous wall segments, to reduce interpreter's variability and augment accuracy." The ASE also suggests using contrast to aid in the diagnosis of pathologies primarily affecting the left ventricular apex such as apical variant of hypertrophic cardiomyopathy, isolated left ventricular noncompaction, apical thrombus, left ventricular aneurysm, or left ventricular pseudoaneurysm. Contrast echocardiography may also be helpful to enhance spectral Doppler signals to evaluate left ventricular diastolic function, hemodynamic assessment, and comprehensive valve evaluations.

Using Contrast Agents for Left Ventricular Opacification

In the United States, two contrast agents have been approved for left ventricular opacification and for endocardial border delineation. These contrast agents are Definity, which has a phospholipid shell, and Optison, which has a shell that is composed of human albumin. When contrast is used for left ventricular opacification, the diagnostic accuracy is enhanced at rest and with stress. This technique is also advantageous for delineation of left ventricular apical anatomy, to confirm pseudoaneurysm, to confirm apical hypertrophy, ventricular noncompaction, and to demonstrate filling defects such as an apical thrombus, etc.

Technique for Left Ventricular Opacification Using Contrast Agents

The technique of left ventricular opacification typically uses harmonic B mode imaging with the mechanical index (MI) set at 0.5. Compression is set in the medium-to-high range with the focus established at the level of the mitral valve or below. An intravenous bolus of contrast is usually the method of administration, but continuous infusion may be used for stress studies. If the MI is too high or the focus is incorrect, apical swirling may occur as a result of increased contrast destruction in the near field. Too much contrast will cause difficulty in visualization of the basal segments.

Using Saline Contrast

In echocardiography, the use of agitated saline contrast is also known as the "bubble test." This test is performed by hand agitation of saline between two 10-ml syringes that are connected to a three-way tap. Five ml of saline and 0.2 ml of air are quickly injected form one syringe to the other until opacity is noted without large visible air bubbles. The air bubbles that result from hand agitation of saline are too big to cross the pulmonary vascular bed; therefore, this technique is useful for visualization of the right heart. A significant amount appearing in the left heart may indicate the presence of an intracardiac shunt.

Performing Continuous-Wave Doppler with a Nonimaging Probe

Continuous-wave Doppler with a nonimaging probe is a technique that is very helpful in the evaluation of aortic stenosis. In fact, studies have suggested that the mean transaortic pressure gradient and peak aortic velocity should be ascertained by using the nonimaging continuous-wave Doppler transducer in numerous views and including the apical and right parasternal views. Nonimaging continuous-wave Doppler yields an optimal alignment with the transaortic valvular jet and enables the recording of the highest velocities, which prevents improper evaluation of the severity of the aortic stenosis.

Harmonic Imaging

Harmonic imaging results in significant improvement in 2D and M-mode image quality. Vibration frequencies that are exact multiples of the fundamental frequency are called harmonics. Ultrasound waves create a high-density compression phase and a low-density refraction phase in tissue. The tissue particles start to oscillate, which results in a fundamental frequency and other vibrations at lower amplitude and higher frequency than the beginning vibrations. Thus, harmonic images can be generated from the nonlinear response. The harmonic aspect of the ultrasound beam gets progressively stronger with the depth of the tissue penetration.

CHANGE POWER OUTPUT

It is important to be familiar with all the controls on the echocardiography imaging agent. It is also crucial to understand how to manipulate the controls to obtain the best image. One such technique is that of changing the power output to enable optimization of the signal-to-noise ratio. Increasing the power output will serve to generate stronger returning echoes as a result of increasing the intensity of the sound beam. It is important to recall, however, that increasing the power output will subsequently result in an increased acoustical exposure for the patient.

How to Overcome Test Anxiety

Just the thought of taking a test is enough to make most people a little nervous. A test is an important event that can have a long-term impact on your future, so it's important to take it seriously and it's natural to feel anxious about performing well. But just because anxiety is normal, that doesn't mean that it's helpful in test taking, or that you should simply accept it as part of your life. Anxiety can have a variety of effects. These effects can be mild, like making you feel slightly nervous, or severe, like blocking your ability to focus or remember even a simple detail.

If you experience test anxiety—whether severe or mild—it's important to know how to beat it. To discover this, first you need to understand what causes test anxiety.

Causes of Test Anxiety

While we often think of anxiety as an uncontrollable emotional state, it can actually be caused by simple, practical things. One of the most common causes of test anxiety is that a person does not feel adequately prepared for their test. This feeling can be the result of many different issues such as poor study habits or lack of organization, but the most common culprit is time management. Starting to study too late, failing to organize your study time to cover all of the material, or being distracted while you study will mean that you're not well prepared for the test. This may lead to cramming the night before, which will cause you to be physically and mentally exhausted for the test. Poor time management also contributes to feelings of stress, fear, and hopelessness as you realize you are not well prepared but don't know what to do about it.

Other times, test anxiety is not related to your preparation for the test but comes from unresolved fear. This may be a past failure on a test, or poor performance on tests in general. It may come from comparing yourself to others who seem to be performing better or from the stress of living up to expectations. Anxiety may be driven by fears of the future—how failure on this test would affect your educational and career goals. These fears are often completely irrational, but they can still negatively impact your test performance.

Elements of Test Anxiety

As mentioned earlier, test anxiety is considered to be an emotional state, but it has physical and mental components as well. Sometimes you may not even realize that you are suffering from test anxiety until you notice the physical symptoms. These can include trembling hands, rapid heartbeat, sweating, nausea, and tense muscles. Extreme anxiety may lead to fainting or vomiting. Obviously, any of these symptoms can have a negative impact on testing. It is important to recognize them as soon as they begin to occur so that you can address the problem before it damages your performance.

The mental components of test anxiety include trouble focusing and inability to remember learned information. During a test, your mind is on high alert, which can help you recall information and stay focused for an extended period of time. However, anxiety interferes with your mind's natural processes, causing you to blank out, even on the questions you know well. The strain of testing during anxiety makes it difficult to stay focused, especially on a test that may take several hours. Extreme anxiety can take a huge mental toll, making it difficult not only to recall test information but even to understand the test questions or pull your thoughts together.

Effects of Test Anxiety

Test anxiety is like a disease—if left untreated, it will get progressively worse. Anxiety leads to poor performance, and this reinforces the feelings of fear and failure, which in turn lead to poor performances on subsequent tests. It can grow from a mild nervousness to a crippling condition. If allowed to progress, test anxiety can have a big impact on your schooling, and consequently on your future.

Test anxiety can spread to other parts of your life. Anxiety on tests can become anxiety in any stressful situation, and blanking on a test can turn into panicking in a job situation. But fortunately, you don't have to let anxiety rule your testing and determine your grades. There are a number of relatively simple steps you can take to move past anxiety and function normally on a test and in the rest of life.

Physical Steps for Beating Test Anxiety

While test anxiety is a serious problem, the good news is that it can be overcome. It doesn't have to control your ability to think and remember information. While it may take time, you can begin taking steps today to beat anxiety.

Just as your first hint that you may be struggling with anxiety comes from the physical symptoms, the first step to treating it is also physical. Rest is crucial for having a clear, strong mind. If you are tired, it is much easier to give in to anxiety. But if you establish good sleep habits, your body and mind will be ready to perform optimally, without the strain of exhaustion. Additionally, sleeping well helps you to retain information better, so you're more likely to recall the answers when you see the test questions.

Getting good sleep means more than going to bed on time. It's important to allow your brain time to relax. Take study breaks from time to time so it doesn't get overworked, and don't study right before bed. Take time to rest your mind before trying to rest your body, or you may find it difficult to fall asleep.

Along with sleep, other aspects of physical health are important in preparing for a test. Good nutrition is vital for good brain function. Sugary foods and drinks may give a burst of energy but this burst is followed by a crash, both physically and emotionally. Instead, fuel your body with protein and vitamin-rich foods.

Also, drink plenty of water. Dehydration can lead to headaches and exhaustion, especially if your brain is already under stress from the rigors of the test. Particularly if your test is a long one, drink water during the breaks. And if possible, take an energy-boosting snack to eat between sections.

Along with sleep and diet, a third important part of physical health is exercise. Maintaining a steady workout schedule is helpful, but even taking 5-minute study breaks to walk can help get your blood pumping faster and clear your head. Exercise also releases endorphins, which contribute to a positive feeling and can help combat test anxiety.

When you nurture your physical health, you are also contributing to your mental health. If your body is healthy, your mind is much more likely to be healthy as well. So take time to rest, nourish your body with healthy food and water, and get moving as much as possible. Taking these physical steps will make you stronger and more able to take the mental steps necessary to overcome test anxiety.

Mental Steps for Beating Test Anxiety

Working on the mental side of test anxiety can be more challenging, but as with the physical side, there are clear steps you can take to overcome it. As mentioned earlier, test anxiety often stems from lack of preparation, so the obvious solution is to prepare for the test. Effective studying may be the most important weapon you have for beating test anxiety, but you can and should employ several other mental tools to combat fear.

First, boost your confidence by reminding yourself of past success—tests or projects that you aced. If you're putting as much effort into preparing for this test as you did for those, there's no reason you should expect to fail here. Work hard to prepare; then trust your preparation.

Second, surround yourself with encouraging people. It can be helpful to find a study group, but be sure that the people you're around will encourage a positive attitude. If you spend time with others who are anxious or cynical, this will only contribute to your own anxiety. Look for others who are motivated to study hard from a desire to succeed, not from a fear of failure.

Third, reward yourself. A test is physically and mentally tiring, even without anxiety, and it can be helpful to have something to look forward to. Plan an activity following the test, regardless of the outcome, such as going to a movie or getting ice cream.

When you are taking the test, if you find yourself beginning to feel anxious, remind yourself that you know the material. Visualize successfully completing the test. Then take a few deep, relaxing breaths and return to it. Work through the questions carefully but with confidence, knowing that you are capable of succeeding.

Developing a healthy mental approach to test taking will also aid in other areas of life. Test anxiety affects more than just the actual test—it can be damaging to your mental health and even contribute to depression. It's important to beat test anxiety before it becomes a problem for more than testing.

Study Strategy

Being prepared for the test is necessary to combat anxiety, but what does being prepared look like? You may study for hours on end and still not feel prepared. What you need is a strategy for test prep. The next few pages outline our recommended steps to help you plan out and conquer the challenge of preparation.

Step 1: Scope Out the Test

Learn everything you can about the format (multiple choice, essay, etc.) and what will be on the test. Gather any study materials, course outlines, or sample exams that may be available. Not only will this help you to prepare, but knowing what to expect can help to alleviate test anxiety.

Step 2: Map Out the Material

Look through the textbook or study guide and make note of how many chapters or sections it has. Then divide these over the time you have. For example, if a book has 15 chapters and you have five days to study, you need to cover three chapters each day. Even better, if you have the time, leave an extra day at the end for overall review after you have gone through the material in depth.

If time is limited, you may need to prioritize the material. Look through it and make note of which sections you think you already have a good grasp on, and which need review. While you are studying, skim quickly through the familiar sections and take more time on the challenging parts. Write out your plan so you don't get lost as you go. Having a written plan also helps you feel more in control of the study, so anxiety is less likely to arise from feeling overwhelmed at the amount to cover.

Step 3: Gather Your Tools

Decide what study method works best for you. Do you prefer to highlight in the book as you study and then go back over the highlighted portions? Or do you type out notes of the important information? Or is it helpful to make flashcards that you can carry with you? Assemble the pens, index cards, highlighters, post-it notes, and any other materials you may need so you won't be distracted by getting up to find things while you study.

If you're having a hard time retaining the information or organizing your notes, experiment with different methods. For example, try color-coding by subject with colored pens, highlighters, or post-it notes. If you learn better by hearing, try recording yourself reading your notes so you can listen while in the car, working out, or simply sitting at your desk. Ask a friend to quiz you from your flashcards, or try teaching someone the material to solidify it in your mind.

Step 4: Create Your Environment

It's important to avoid distractions while you study. This includes both the obvious distractions like visitors and the subtle distractions like an uncomfortable chair (or a too-comfortable couch that makes you want to fall asleep). Set up the best study environment possible: good lighting and a comfortable work area. If background music helps you focus, you may want to turn it on, but otherwise keep the room quiet. If you are using a computer to take notes, be sure you don't have any other windows open, especially applications like social media, games, or anything else that could distract you. Silence your phone and turn off notifications. Be sure to keep water close by so you stay hydrated while you study (but avoid unhealthy drinks and snacks).

Also, take into account the best time of day to study. Are you freshest first thing in the morning? Try to set aside some time then to work through the material. Is your mind clearer in the afternoon or evening? Schedule your study session then. Another method is to study at the same time of day that you will take the test, so that your brain gets used to working on the material at that time and will be ready to focus at test time.

Step 5: Study!

Once you have done all the study preparation, it's time to settle into the actual studying. Sit down, take a few moments to settle your mind so you can focus, and begin to follow your study plan. Don't give in to distractions or let yourself procrastinate. This is your time to prepare so you'll be ready to fearlessly approach the test. Make the most of the time and stay focused.

Of course, you don't want to burn out. If you study too long you may find that you're not retaining the information very well. Take regular study breaks. For example, taking five minutes out of every hour to walk briskly, breathing deeply and swinging your arms, can help your mind stay fresh.

As you get to the end of each chapter or section, it's a good idea to do a quick review. Remind yourself of what you learned and work on any difficult parts. When you feel that you've mastered the material, move on to the next part. At the end of your study session, briefly skim through your notes again.

But while review is helpful, cramming last minute is NOT. If at all possible, work ahead so that you won't need to fit all your study into the last day. Cramming overloads your brain with more information than it can process and retain, and your tired mind may struggle to recall even previously learned information when it is overwhelmed with last-minute study. Also, the urgent nature of cramming and the stress placed on your brain contribute to anxiety. You'll be more likely to go to the test feeling unprepared and having trouble thinking clearly.

So don't cram, and don't stay up late before the test, even just to review your notes at a leisurely pace. Your brain needs rest more than it needs to go over the information again. In fact, plan to finish your studies by noon or early afternoon the day before the test. Give your brain the rest of the day to relax or focus on other things, and get a good night's sleep. Then you will be fresh for the test and better able to recall what you've studied.

Step 6: Take a Practice Test

Many courses offer sample tests, either online or in the study materials. This is an excellent resource to check whether you have mastered the material, as well as to prepare for the test format and environment.

Check the test format ahead of time: the number of questions, the type (multiple choice, free response, etc.), and the time limit. Then create a plan for working through them. For example, if you have 30 minutes to take a 60-question test, your limit is 30 seconds per question. Spend less time on the questions you know well so that you can take more time on the difficult ones.

If you have time to take several practice tests, take the first one open book, with no time limit. Work through the questions at your own pace and make sure you fully understand them. Gradually work up to taking a test under test conditions: sit at a desk with all study materials put away and set a timer. Pace yourself to make sure you finish the test with time to spare and go back to check your answers if you have time.

After each test, check your answers. On the questions you missed, be sure you understand why you missed them. Did you misread the question (tests can use tricky wording)? Did you forget the information? Or was it something you hadn't learned? Go back and study any shaky areas that the practice tests reveal.

Taking these tests not only helps with your grade, but also aids in combating test anxiety. If you're already used to the test conditions, you're less likely to worry about it, and working through tests until you're scoring well gives you a confidence boost. Go through the practice tests until you feel comfortable, and then you can go into the test knowing that you're ready for it.

Test Tips

On test day, you should be confident, knowing that you've prepared well and are ready to answer the questions. But aside from preparation, there are several test day strategies you can employ to maximize your performance.

First, as stated before, get a good night's sleep the night before the test (and for several nights before that, if possible). Go into the test with a fresh, alert mind rather than staying up late to study.

Try not to change too much about your normal routine on the day of the test. It's important to eat a nutritious breakfast, but if you normally don't eat breakfast at all, consider eating just a protein bar. If you're a coffee drinker, go ahead and have your normal coffee. Just make sure you time it so that the caffeine doesn't wear off right in the middle of your test. Avoid sugary beverages, and drink enough water to stay hydrated but not so much that you need a restroom break 10 minutes into the test. If your test isn't first thing in the morning, consider going for a walk or doing a light workout before the test to get your blood flowing.

Allow yourself enough time to get ready, and leave for the test with plenty of time to spare so you won't have the anxiety of scrambling to arrive in time. Another reason to be early is to select a good seat. It's helpful to sit away from doors and windows, which can be distracting. Find a good seat, get out your supplies, and settle your mind before the test begins.

When the test begins, start by going over the instructions carefully, even if you already know what to expect. Make sure you avoid any careless mistakes by following the directions.

Then begin working through the questions, pacing yourself as you've practiced. If you're not sure on an answer, don't spend too much time on it, and don't let it shake your confidence. Either skip it and come back later, or eliminate as many wrong answers as possible and guess among the remaining ones. Don't dwell on these questions as you continue—put them out of your mind and focus on what lies ahead.

Be sure to read all of the answer choices, even if you're sure the first one is the right answer. Sometimes you'll find a better one if you keep reading. But don't second-guess yourself if you do immediately know the answer. Your gut instinct is usually right. Don't let test anxiety rob you of the information you know.

If you have time at the end of the test (and if the test format allows), go back and review your answers. Be cautious about changing any, since your first instinct tends to be correct, but make sure you didn't misread any of the questions or accidentally mark the wrong answer choice. Look over any you skipped and make an educated guess.

At the end, leave the test feeling confident. You've done your best, so don't waste time worrying about your performance or wishing you could change anything. Instead, celebrate the successful completion of this test. And finally, use this test to learn how to deal with anxiety even better next time.

Review Video: Test Anxiety
Visit mometrix.com/academy and enter code: 100340

Important Qualification

Not all anxiety is created equal. If your test anxiety is causing major issues in your life beyond the classroom or testing center, or if you are experiencing troubling physical symptoms related to your anxiety, it may be a sign of a serious physiological or psychological condition. If this sounds like your situation, we strongly encourage you to seek professional help.

Online Resources

Due to our efforts to try to keep this book to a manageable length, we've created a link that will give you access to all of your online resources:

mometrix.com/resources719/ardmsadultec

It's Your Moment, Let's Celebrate It!

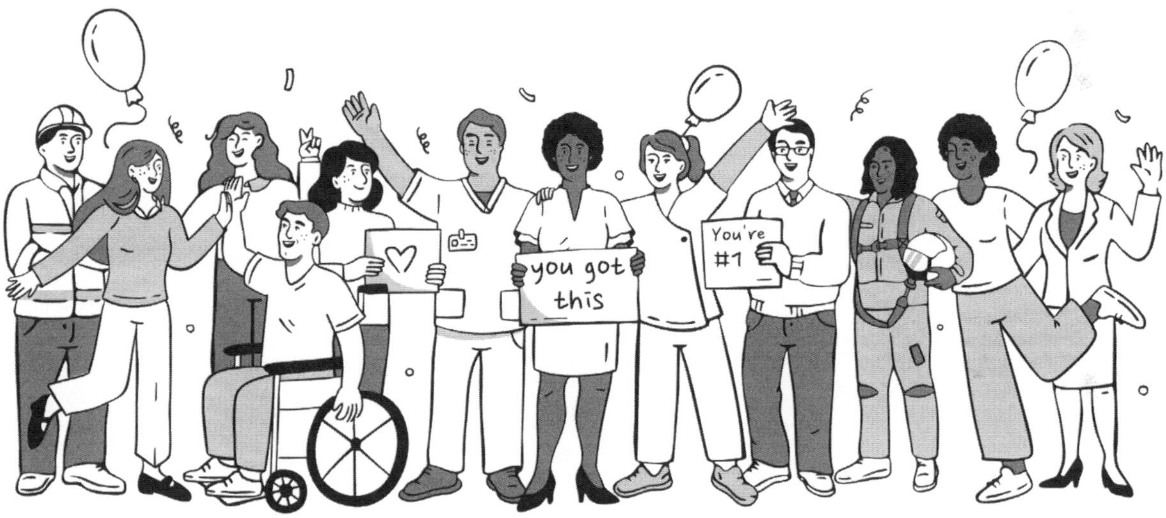

Share your story @mometrixtestpreparation